# FLUENCY PLUS

MANAGING FLUENCY DISORDERS IN INDIVIDUALS WITH MULTIPLE DIAGNOSES

# FLUENCY PLUS

MANAGING FLUENCY DISORDERS IN INDIVIDUALS WITH MULTIPLE DIAGNOSES

*Kathleen Scaler Scott, PhD, CCC-SLP, BCS-F*

Misericordia University

Dallas, Pennsylvania

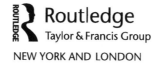

Routledge

Taylor & Francis Group

NEW YORK AND LONDON

*Fluency Plus: Managing Fluency Disorders in Individuals With Multiple Diagnoses* includes ancillary materials specifically available for faculty use. Included are PowerPoint slides. Please visit www.routledge.com/9781630913106.

First published in 2018 by SLACK Incorporated

Published in 2024 by Routledge
605 Third Avenue, New York, NY 10158

and by Routledge
4 Park Square, Milton Park, Abingdon, Oxon, OX14 4RN

*Routledge is an imprint of the Taylor & Francis Group, an informa business*

© 2018 Taylor & Francis Group

*Dr. Kathleen Scaler Scott* has no financial or proprietary interest in the materials presented herein.

*Trademark notice*: Product or corporate names may be trademarks or registered trademarks, and are used only for identification and explanation without intent to infringe.

Cover Artist: Anita Santiago

Library of Congress Cataloging-in-Publication Data

Names: Scott, Kathleen Scaler, 1969- author.
Title: Fluency plus : managing fluency disorders in individuals with multiple
  diagnoses / Kathleen Scaler Scott.
Description: Thorofare, NJ : SLACK Incorporated, [2018] | Includes
  bibliographical references and index.
Identifiers: LCCN 2018015062 (print) |
  | ISBN 9781630913106
  (paperback : alk. paper)
Subjects: | MESH: Speech Therapy--methods | Speech Disorders--therapy |
  Speech Disorders--complications | Neurodevelopmental
  Disorders--complications | Evidence-Based Practice
Classification: LCC RC428.8 (print) | NLM WL 340.3 |
  DDC 616.85/506--dc23
LC record available at https://lccn.loc.gov/2018015062


ISBN: 9781630913106 (pbk)
ISBN: 9781003524199 (ebk)


DOI: 10.4324/9781003524199

# DEDICATION

To my mom:
If I ever get a "sister," I want one just like you.


To my husband:
You've embraced all the sacrifices that come with this crazy life,
and to you I am forever grateful.

# CONTENTS

# ACKNOWLEDGMENTS

I wish to thank the many people who made this book possible. I am sincerely grateful to all of my students and colleagues at Misericordia University, who encouraged and inspired me to keep moving forward on a daily basis. To my former student, Sarah Tokach, who walked alongside me this entire project and provided meaningful feedback on each chapter, thank you. I appreciate everything you bring to this world and the support you've brought me. I am proud to call you my colleague. To my editor, Brien Cummings, who supported me from initial brainstorming of how to make an idea become reality all the way through to production, I am forever grateful. He endured, with constant patience and encouragement, the long delays that happened as life got in the way. Thank you. Thanks to the SLACK Incorporated production team for their steadfast commitment to all stages of this project. To all the pioneers in fluency disorders who came before me, instilled me with knowledge, and inspired me to share my passion with others, thank you for your leadership and generosity. To the colleagues from clinical, research, and academic settings who I consider mentors along my professional journey: Mary Ann Raymond, Sue Stephens, Marlene Stankus, Terri Rossman, Deborah Peters, Scott Yaruss, John Tetnowski, Ken St. Louis, Flo Myers, Klaas Bakker, Larry Raphael, David Ward, and Glen Tellis. Thank you for all you've taught me about being a clinician, academic, and researcher. Finally, thanks to all clients and families who continue to teach me every day that there is always more to learn.

# ABOUT THE AUTHOR

*Kathleen Scaler Scott, PhD, CCC-SLP, BCS-F,* is a practicing speech-language pathologist, board-certified specialist in fluency disorders, and associate professor of speech-language pathology at Misericordia University in Dallas, Pennsylvania. She has been a practicing clinician for over 25 years in school, hospital, and private practice settings. Her clinical and research work has included focus on the impact of executive functions on daily speech and communication. Dr. Scaler Scott's research interests are largely in cluttering, atypical disfluency, and clinician training and treatment effectiveness. She is the co-editor of *Cluttering: A Handbook of Research, Intervention, and Education* (2011) and co-author of *Managing Cluttering: A Comprehensive Guidebook of Activities* (2013), both with Dr. David Ward. Dr. Scaler Scott has spoken nationally and internationally on the topics of fluency and social pragmatic disorders. She is a certified special education and elementary education teacher and was the first coordinator of the International Cluttering Association.

# PREFACE

When I am given meaningful advice, I often think this about the advice giver: "They get it." To give advice that is truly meaningful, you need to have shared a similar experience with the person you are advising. I have found that the most meaningful advice I've gotten about enjoying the experience of my wedding came from someone who had experienced their own. Likewise, the most meaningful advice about being a caregiver for a mother with dementia came from those caregivers who wore the battle scars reflected in their exhausted faces, bodies, and tone of voice. If I weren't still in the trenches as a practicing clinician on a daily basis, treating clients with all fluency disorders and every concomitant diagnosis represented in this book, I'm not sure I'd feel myself qualified to write this book. I've been in the trenches in schools, hospitals, and private practice. Because I've wrestled with heavy caseloads, knowledgeable parents and clients who ask lots of questions, and increasingly complex disorders, I've been and continue to be challenged in many ways. I've had to figure out the best ways to understand the populations I'm dealing with; structure my sessions to get the most out of a client in a short amount of time; and create sessions and home activities that are functional, practical, and doable for busy families.

As speech-language pathologists, students, researchers, and academics, there are days when we feel like the professional demands on us are endless. As I write this, the emails are flowing in with new demands that overtake the original to-do list. It is my hope that *Fluency Plus: Managing Fluency Disorders in Individuals With Multiple Diagnoses* will bring you a streamlined and straightforward approach to assisting clients with multiple needs. Although the names have been changed for confidentiality, the case studies throughout the book are the stories of clients I've worked with who have pushed me outside my comfort zone in terms of professional advancement. They represent only a small fraction of clients who have driven me to seek new information from multiple disciplines and incorporate this information into daily practice. They've pushed me to test hypotheses, moving forward when things work out, and readjusting when they do not.

In sharing the stories and information I've gleaned with you, my hope is to provide you with meaningful information. Meaningful to me means the information is accessible yet challenging for all levels of clinical training and education. Meaningful means the information provides a foundation from which you can feel comfortable problem solving assessment and treatment decisions. Meaningful means clinicians can take the activities and adapt them to multiple clients and work contexts. Most of all, meaningful means that when you read this book I have conveyed my awareness of the realities of a day-to-day caseload and how there are so many factors to consider other than the initial diagnosis. I hope when you read this you think, "She gets it." I will never have gotten it all, but every day I strive to "get it" more. I hope you do, too.

# CHAPTER 1

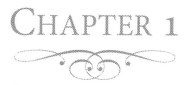

# INTRODUCTION

## HISTORY

Twenty-five years ago, while working as a speech-language clinician at a school for children with learning differences, I came upon my first client with cluttering. At first I did not know that the appropriate diagnosis was cluttering. I only knew that this client was not stuttering and that there was something more. My newly completed master's degree had prepared me to work with the client's language and literacy skills. Colleagues and continuing education in my new work setting helped me to understand and plan for the client's additional diagnosis of attention deficit hyperactivity disorder (ADHD). However, my graduate coursework had offered no information on cluttering. My own research led me to one clinically-based journal article about cluttering. I relied heavily upon this article to identify and treat the cluttering. It was a challenge to add cluttering goals to the client's already long list of goals in his individualized education program (IEP). But even more of a challenge was how to help a child with ADHD, who already had difficulty with self-regulation, do what he needed to do to manage his cluttering: regulate the rate of his speech.

Seven years later, while working with a teen with articulation and pragmatic difficulties, I listened as I heard another type of disfluency that was not stuttering. This child exhibited word-final disfluencies (WFDs). Again, my academic and clinical training had not prepared me to work with this disorder. I found some research on the phenomenon, but no published clinical strategies.

Five years later, I began my doctoral studies in fluency disorders. My goal in getting this degree was to gain the research skills needed to conduct further study of WFDs and cluttering. My ultimate goal was to provide evidence-based treatment strategies to the clinicians working with these clients. As a doctoral student, a colleague and I conducted one workshop regarding disfluencies in autism spectrum disorders at a national convention. The session was packed, and afterward, the email questions began to overtake our inboxes. More and more clinicians were asking, "Is my client cluttering?" "I hear these disfluencies that are not stuttering but am not sure what they are. What do I do? How do I evaluate/ treat them?"

Scaler Scott, K.
*Fluency Plus: Managing Fluency Disorders in
Individuals With Multiple Diagnoses (pp 1–4).*
© 2018 Taylor & Francis Group.

The growing need among speech-language pathologists for more information about these fluency disorders has become increasingly clear to me in more recent years. What also became clear was what I found in the details of these email questions. The majority of the time, when a speech-language clinician described a client with a "different" type of fluency disorder, they also described a client who had additional diagnoses to contend with, such as autism, ADHD, childhood apraxia of speech, learning disabilities, severe articulation and/or phonological disorders, intellectual disability, and/or selective mutism. As students and practicing clinicians are being asked to see more complex cases, the training needs are becoming more complex. I note this same trend of "fluency plus" other diagnoses as part of my current role as associate professor and clinical supervisor in a university speech-language pathology program. Long ago and far away are the days when clinicians are being asked to see a client with just one disorder. Most days when graduate students are bringing their fluency cases to me for review, there are other issues to contend with. I am now known in our university clinic as the supervisor for "fluency plus" cases.

*Long ago and far away are the days when clinicians are being asked to see a client with just one disorder.*

The body of research we have on cluttering within the past 10 to 15 years is growing stronger with each completed study. Though not perfect, definition of the disorder and research methodology is becoming tighter, allowing consumers of the research to draw more conclusions than in the past, when the diagnoses of the study's participants were not clearly defined. We are also gaining ground on the research on WFDs. I strive to contribute to this growing body of research, and the name of my university research team has also become known as the "fluency plus" team.

# PURPOSE

I just took you through my career history to demonstrate that this book is written from multiple perspectives. You'll see in that story that I was a clinician first and a professional who needed more information to best help her clients. As a practicing clinician, each day I am testing treatments based upon the current evidence. Real-life experience teaches me what works only in theory and what works in everyday clinical practice. As an active researcher and professor, I am providing students and clinicians with the needed background information to understand what we currently do and do not know in the field of "fluency plus" disorders. As a clinical supervisor, I am asked to suggest practical strategies for applying what we do know to daily clinical practice. As a faculty member who teaches a full load of coursework, I am always striving to provide content that is accessible for both undergraduate and graduate students in a speech-language pathology program, as well as supplemental materials that can be used by a busy lecturer and/or clinical supervisor.

As a practicing clinician, clinical supervisor, and faculty member, I understand where the needs of each of these groups overlap and where they may differ slightly. This book is therefore designed to provide the most up-to-date research, clinical applications, and specific clinical activities to incorporate into daily practice. It is written so that the content is within reach of students, practicing clinicians, and faculty alike.

# How to Use This Book

How the reader uses this book may vary based on need. For example, should this book be used as part of a fluency or other communication disorders class, faculty may find using the book in order from beginning to end will provide students the best perspective of fluency and concomitant disorders. Faculty may also find the case studies woven throughout the book and the online supplemental content instructor materials (which include PowerPoint slides for each chapter) useful for designing classroom content. Should this book be used in a university or off-campus clinic, student clinicians will gain thorough background knowledge from Chapters 2 through 4. They can then select the relevant chapter(s) focusing specifically on the concomitant disorder(s) they are treating. Principles of how to work with fluency and concomitant disorders is the focus of Chapter 3, and Chapters 5 through 11 provide specifics about disorders commonly associated with fluency disorders. After background information is gained on fluency disorders and principles for working with concomitant disorders

*This book is designed to provide the most up-to-date research, clinical applications, and specific clinical activities to incorporate into daily practice. It is written on a level so that the content is within reach of students, practicing clinicians, and faculty alike.*

in previous chapters, the chapters on specific disorders can stand alone and do not need to be read in a particular order. Practicing clinicians and/or those training practicing clinicians, whether fluency specialists or not, will find clinical tips and reminders throughout the book. Those who have limited experience with fluency disorders, such as students, new clinicians, and clinicians with a low incidence of fluency disorders on their caseloads, will gain necessary background knowledge on identifying and differentially diagnosing various fluency disorders and an overview of treatment strategies in Chapter 2. All readers will find a summary of the latest information related to fluency disorders and executive functioning, and practical implications of this information, in Chapter 4.

# Content and Organization

Chapters 2 through 4 are meant to provide the reader with comprehensive background information on 1) defining stuttering, cluttering, and other atypical disfluencies; 2) understanding the current state of the research regarding assessment, differential diagnosis, and treatment of these disorders; 3) factors to consider when working with fluency and concomitant disorders; and 4) understanding executive functioning and how it relates to planning treatment for these cases. Chapters 5 through 11 focus on "fluency plus" specific accompanying disorders. Each of the these chapters contains the following sections:

- Fluency concerns most commonly identified in this population
- Fluency treatment myths and facts in this population
- Executive functioning challenges expected in this population
- Clinical management strategies
- Self-regulation strategies and activities
- Treatment activities

Finally, Chapter 12 provides the clinician with some parting strategies to keep in mind in daily problem solving while working with the "fluency plus" population. Perhaps you've come to this book because you first were interested in fluency and gradually noticed the clients you are treating, supervising, and/or teaching about are broadening in terms of needs. Or perhaps you started with your interest in another area, such as language or autism, only to find that the clients you are treating, supervising, and/or teaching about also have fluency concerns. Perhaps you are a clinician working in a busy school and see more and more clients with overlapping needs. Perhaps you are a student in speech-language pathology wondering about fluency concerns that are different from what you know as stuttering. No matter which way you arrived at this book, I hope that the journey through it will help you feel better equipped to address all of your clients' communication needs.

# CHAPTER 2

# BACKGROUND, TERMS, DEFINITIONS, AND STATE OF THE RESEARCH

Stuttering, cluttering, and other disfluencies may occur separately or together in a single client. Stuttering is easily identified by name among the public. There is also some ability among the public to identify people with cluttering, given a definition (St. Louis et al., 2010). Atypical disfluencies are increasingly identified by clinicians, though not as consistently by the layperson. When clinicians do identify atypical disfluencies, this often comes with a myriad of questions they cannot answer, including questions related to concomitant disorders. This chapter will attempt to clarify the difference between stuttering, cluttering, and atypical disfluencies, and to provide a framework for evaluation and differential diagnosis.

## DEFINITIONS

### Stuttering

Although there is no universally agreed upon definition of stuttering, there is enough consensus to make research and clinical work with this population fairly straightforward. For the purposes of this book, stuttering will be defined as speech hesitations that keep a speaker from moving forward. These hesitations are not related to the client being unclear about their message. The speaker who is only stuttering is clear about their message but has trouble moving forward to produce the sounds that make up the message. The difficulties are typically seen in one of four physical symptoms: 1) repetitions of sounds or syllables (e.g., "p-p-parent" or "bi-bi-bicycle"); 2) tense repetition of single-syllable words (e.g., "I-I-I"); 3) prolongations of sounds (e.g., "sssunshine" or "suuuunshine"); and 4) blocks, whereby a client becomes stuck on a specific sound and there is either silence or audible attempts at producing the sound. These symptoms are known as stuttering-like disfluencies (SLDs; Ambrose & Yairi, 1999; Yairi & Ambrose, 1992). The client may also experience other physical symptoms, which can reflect underlying tension or struggle, such as eye blinking, fist squeezing, or foot stomping. These symptoms are known as secondary behaviors and are thought to be classically conditioned when a client first uses them (whether with conscious knowledge of their use or not) to avoid or escape a moment of stuttering

Scaler Scott, K.
*Fluency Plus: Managing Fluency Disorders in Individuals With Multiple Diagnoses (pp 5–34).*
© 2018 Taylor & Francis Group.

(Brutten & Shoemaker, 1967). Physical symptoms combined with secondary behaviors are known as the behavioral components of stuttering. In addition to the physical symptoms of stuttering, it is well recognized that stuttering can have a negative life impact upon some clients. This negative impact includes feelings and thoughts the client may have about their stuttering that can in turn affect their communication behavior. For example, a client may feel ashamed of their stuttering, which may lead to switching words to avoid stuttering or failing to participate in a class discussion. The thoughts may include client perceptions of how stuttering affects their life. Such thoughts may include, "If I say my name, I'll stutter," or "I can't get promoted because I stutter." At times these perceptions are based upon real lived experiences (e.g., the client has frequently stuttered when they've said their name), whereas at other times they may be based upon the client's perception of what they believe will happen to them (e.g., the client has not applied for a promotion because they feel they will not receive it due to stuttering). If a client believes that each time they say their name, they may stutter, they may avoid introducing themselves, change their name, or put a filler word before their introduction to help them get started (e.g., "My name is uh Jim"). The feelings a client experiences are known as the affective components of stuttering, and the thoughts are known as the cognitive components of stuttering (Yaruss & Quesal, 2006). Different clients experience varying degrees of behavioral, affective, and cognitive components of stuttering. In extreme cases, a client may experience such negative affective and/or cognitive components that she or he will hide all stuttering. Hiding can mean that the client constantly engages in word changing, talks significantly less than they normally would, and/or doesn't let others know they stutter. When stuttering is hidden, it is known as covert stuttering. There are varying degrees of covert stuttering. For example, a client may hide their stuttering from everyone, including close family, or from everyone except close family. Because of the serious negative impact the affective and cognitive components can have upon overall communication, stuttering evaluations are incomplete if the affective, behavioral, and cognitive components are not all thoroughly explored. There are some clients who exhibit no outward symptoms of stuttering yet engage in continuous avoidance. Although the avoidance behaviors may not be evident to the casual observer, the consequences of these behaviors are quite significant for the client and have their roots in the stuttering disorder. Therefore, outward symptoms of stuttering need not always be present for a client to be diagnosed with a stuttering disorder. Conversely, some clients present with many overt stuttering behaviors (repetitions, prolongations, and/ or blocks) yet feel no negative impact of these behaviors upon their communication. Therefore, outward symptoms of stuttering do not always confirm the true impact of a stuttering disorder and whether or not the observed stuttering behaviors require treatment. Designing treatment individualized to client needs based upon their symptoms of stuttering will be emphasized throughout this book.

## Cluttering

Cluttering is a communication disorder that has a long history in the field of fluency disorders. In that history, cluttering's definition has changed numerous times (Table 2-1). Professionals most commonly identify rapid rate and excessive disfluencies (St. Louis, 1996) as agreed upon symptoms of cluttering. Yet what other symptoms exist beyond these two has frequently been debated.

Although descriptions of cluttering have been documented for 300 years, Deso Weiss produced the first published book on the topic in 1964. The book provided a broad definition of cluttering. Weiss painted a picture of a client who not only had difficulty with clarity of speech, but also exhibited other symptoms. Such symptoms included impulsivity, pragmatic, and motor difficulties. In this way, cluttering was described more like a syndrome than a specific communication disorder. Over time, the definition changed shape and added and subtracted symptoms, but always included symptoms other than speech (e.g., motor, pragmatic). Because the definition was so open, clinicians found it difficult to definitively determine whether their client(s) were actually cluttering or whether their behaviors were

| TABLE 2-1 | | |
| :---: | :---: | :---: |
| **Changing Symptoms Included in the Definition of Cluttering** | | |
| *TIME PERIOD* | *AUTHOR(S)* | *FEATURES* |
| 1964 | Deso Weis | "Central language imbalance": messy, impulsive, pragmatic difficulties, difficult to understand and follow speech |
| 1987 | American Psychiatric Association for Diagnostic and Statistical Manual of Mental Disorders, Third Edition—Revised | Definition included lack of awareness |
| 1992 | World Health Organization | Definition included rate, phrasing, disfluency |
| 1999 | American Speech-Language Hearing Association Special Interest Committee | Definition included associated phonological, language, attention symptoms |
| 1992; 2007 | St. Louis; St. Louis, Myers, Bakker, & Raphael | Beginnings of lowest common denominator definition |
| 2006a, 2006b | Daly & Cantrell | Impairments can occur in four areas: pragmatics, speech-motor, language-cognition, motor coordination-writing |
| 2011 | St. Louis & Schulte | Lowest common denominator: symptoms focused only on rate, fluency, rhythm, and clarity |

linked to a concomitant disorder. For example, many of the pragmatic symptoms included in cluttering might also be linked to autism or learning disabilities. Did this mean that all children with autism or learning disabilities were clutterers? What symptoms were mandatory for a diagnosis of cluttering? How do we differentiate those symptoms from symptoms of other disorders? Confusion grew among clinicians and researchers regarding what cluttering was and was not. Because there was no clear definition of cluttering, the concept that cluttering even existed as its own disorder fell out of favor with a lot of clinicians and researchers (St. Louis, Myers, Bakker, & Raphael, 2007), particularly in the United States. Many began to view cluttering as stuttering with additional components; others felt that the lack of definition meant there was no true cluttering disorder. Cluttering began to be known as the "orphan" of speech-language pathology (Daly, 1993). Although the disorder was originally "born" to the parent of fluency disorders, it also had foster parents in the areas of language, pragmatics, and articulation. There was no clear home for cluttering.

Although the concept of cluttering may have been rejected by many, practicing clinicians still had questions. Because cluttering was not clearly defined, clinicians had no choice but to identify and treat whatever symptoms had been put forth in previous definitions (e.g., rapid rate, lack of awareness of communication disorder, decreased speech intelligibility, decreased legibility of handwriting). Confusion between stuttering and cluttering and misdiagnosis of cluttering continued. Dr. Kenneth St. Louis first proposed the need for a "lowest common denominator" (LCD) definition of cluttering in 1992. This proposal attempts to scale the definition of cluttering down to the components clinicians most commonly observe when clients are identified to have "cluttered speech." As previously mentioned, the most common symptoms often identified by clinicians are rate and disfluency (St. Louis, 1996). Although the LCD definition acknowledges that many with cluttering may have other symptoms outside of this definition, these symptoms are seen as concomitant to cluttering rather than universally part of cluttering itself. Scaling cluttering diagnosis down to the LCD is based upon the research that, although all those with cluttering have some degree of difficulty with communicating intelligibly, not all those with this core issue universally exhibit other symptoms, such as difficulties with language and/or handwriting (see St. Louis, 1992, for review). St. Louis and colleagues presented several LCD definitions (St. Louis, 1992; St. Louis et al., 2007; St. Louis, Raphael, Myers, & Bakker, 2003). In 2011, St. Louis and Schulte proposed a refined LCD definition based upon a research study with pure clutterers. Schulte conducted a study of 15 people with cluttering between the ages of 9 and 65; these participants were referred by speech-language clinicians in Germany. Clinicians were asked to refer those they thought were cluttering, but not to refer anyone who also exhibited stuttering. Three participants from the original sample of 18 were excluded from the study due to concomitant stuttering. The intent of the study was to determine how well the proposed LCD definition detected cluttering and to determine what percentage of coexisting disorders would be identified in this sample of people with cluttering. Symptoms in the proposed LCD definition were identified in 13 out of 15 participants, or 87% of the sample. The researchers hypothesized that two participants who did not meet the criteria outlined in the LCD definition may have normalized during the study, as this has been found to be a common occurrence in cluttering (St. Louis & Schulte, 2011). Additionally, each one of the 13 participants presented with at least one coexisting disorder. Sixty-nine percent of the participants presented with between one and three coexisting disorders in the areas of auditory processing, attention deficit hyperactivity disorder, writing, or oral motor difficulties. The resulting definition of cluttering (St. Louis & Schulte, 2011) is that which is frequently used in research and clinical work today:

> Cluttering is a fluency disorder wherein segments of conversation[1] in the speaker's native language[2] typically are perceived as too fast overall[3], too irregular[4], or both. The segments of rapid and/or irregular speech rate must further be accompanied by one or more of the following: (a) excessive "normal" disfluencies[5]; (b) excessive collapsing[6] or deletion of syllables; and/or (c) abnormal pauses, syllable stress, or speech rhythm (pp. 241-242).

[1] Cluttering must occur in naturalistic conversation, but it need not occur even a majority of the time. Clear but isolated examples that exceed those observed in normal speakers are sufficient for a diagnosis.

[2] This may also apply to the speaker's mastered and habitual non-native language, especially in multilingual living environments.

[3] This may be true even though syllable rates may not exceed those of normal speakers.

[4] Synonyms for irregular rate include "jerky," or "spurty."

[5] These disfluencies are often observed in smaller numbers in normal speakers and are typically not observed in stuttering.

[6] Collapsing includes, but is not limited to, excessive shortening, "telescoping," or "over-coarticulating" various syllables, especially in multisyllabic words.

It is important to make two points regarding this LCD definition. First, the disfluencies that are listed as "normal disfluencies" refer to what is commonly known in the literature as non–stuttering-like disfluencies (NSLDs; Ambrose & Yairi, 1999; St. Louis & Schulte, 2011; Yairi & Ambrose, 1992). These are the disfluencies that any speaker may experience when formulating ideas, such as phrase repetitions (e.g., "I want, I want to stop at the store"), revisions of thought ("I need milk, no juice"), and/or interjections (e.g., "um, uh, like, er," etc.). Although the disfluencies noted in cluttering are not stuttering-like, they are different from atypical disfluencies, which will be further defined later. Second, the "abnormal pauses, syllable stress, and speech rhythm" (St. Louis & Schulte, 2011, p. 242) are different from the atypical prosodic patterns often exhibited by individuals on the autism spectrum. What is meant by the abnormal pauses is that pauses appear in places where one would not expect them grammatically.

St. Louis and Schulte (2011) also point out that when pauses do occur, they might be longer than expected by the listener, or the pauses might have "other abnormalities" (p. 244). For example, pauses are often placed naturally by the fluent speaker at clause boundaries, such as:

When he gets home (pause) we will have dinner.

For someone who clutters, the pause might be placed somewhere in the phrase not expected in fluent speech. For example:

When he gets (pause) home we will have dinner.

*OR*

When he gets home, we will have (pause) dinner.

The reason for atypical pauses among those with cluttering is unknown. It is reasonable to hypothesize, given the fact that we have evidence that those with cluttering don't use as many pauses in their speech as typical speakers (Myers & St. Louis, 1996; Scaler Scott, Harris, & St. Louis, 2013), that they may run out of breath and require a pause in a place that is awkward grammatically. This area requires further study.

Adopting the LCD definition of cluttering has made the process of evaluation, differential diagnosis, and treatment much more straightforward for the practicing clinician. The full adoption of this definition has been the result of updates in the literature that dispel some of the previous thoughts about cluttering. These will be covered in detail in the "Current State of the Research" section of this chapter. One thing that will be explored further in that section, but bears mentioning now at the time of definition, is that just as sometimes this occurs for people who stutter, some people who clutter also experience negative attitudes and feelings toward communication (Scaler Scott & St. Louis, 2011). Although these components are not part of the current definition of cluttering, they are nonetheless important to evaluate in clients in order to obtain a picture of the full impact of cluttering on a client's overall communication.

## *Atypical Disfluencies*

Atypical disfluency is a term that has been used anecdotally in clinical and academic settings. First use of this term was noted when St. Louis edited a book titled, *The Atypical Stutterer* in 1986. This book focused on subgroups of those who stutter who would warrant special consideration in terms of assessment and treatment. These subgroups included very severe stuttering, women who stutter, people with neurological stuttering, stuttering in those with cultural differences, stuttering in those with mental retardation (now referred to as intellectual disability), psychogenic stuttering, and cluttering. Atypical disfluency currently refers to patterns of disfluency that seem similar to stuttering but may not be stuttering. The term has only recently been used in conference forums. Osborne (2004) was the first to use the term "atypical stuttering" in the literature to describe disfluencies that occurred mostly in the medial position of words. In a study of disfluency in preschoolers with autism, Plexico, Cleary, McAlpine, and Plumb (2010) categorized disfluencies that included final-sound repetitions (animal-mal) and prolongations (glassss), broken words (op_e_n), and mid-word insertions (straw-da-berry) as atypical disfluencies (p. 45). Scaler Scott et al. (2014) used a similar categorization in a study of disfluency in school-aged children with autism, children who stutter, and controls, but included only word-final repetitions (e.g., "light-t", "light-ight") and prolongations (e.g., "thissss") in this categorization. Sisskin and Wasilus (2014) were the first to define the term atypical disfluencies formally in the literature. Their definition includes word-medial repetitions (e.g., ba-a-a-a-ck"), prolongations (e.g., baaaack), and sound insertions (e.g., "ri—uh—ce") and word-final repetitions, prolongations, and blocks. Prior to this formal definition, one type of atypical disfluency, word-final disfluency (WFD), had been documented in the literature since 1984. Rudmin (1984) documented the WFDs in a young preschooler with no other speech-language issues except initial stuttering-like prolongations. The majority of the time these WFDs have been documented, they have been associated with some other diagnosis. The diagnoses have included those that would fit under the category of developmental disorders such as autism (MacMillan, Kokolakis, Sheedy, & Packman, 2014; Plexico et al., 2010; Scaler Scott, Sutkowski, Tokach, & Leiman, 2015; Scaler Scott, Tetnowski, Flaitz, & Yaruss, 2014; Scott, Grossman, Abendroth, Tetnowski, & Damico, 2006; Sisskin, 2006; Sisskin & Wasilus, 2014; Tetnowski, Richels, Shenker, Sisskin, & Wolk, 2012), Down syndrome (Lebrun & Van Borsel, 1990; Stansfield, 1995), and other disorders accompanied by intellectual disability (Stansfield, 1995). They have also been found in learning disabilities (Lebrun & Van Borsel, 1990) and psychological disorders such as attention deficit hyperactivity disorder (Scaler Scott et. al., 2015; Tetnowski, Scaler Scott, Grossman, Abendroth, & Damico, 2006) and anxiety (MacMillan et al., 2014) and neurological disorders such as neurofibromatosis (Cosyns et al., 2010; Cosyns, Mortier, Corthals, Janssens, & Van Borsel, 2010), Prader-Willi syndrome, and Tourette syndrome (Van Borsel & Tetnowski, 2007). The disfluencies have also been documented in children with no other diagnosis (Camarata, 1989; McAllister & Kingston, 1995; Mowrer, 1987; Rudmin, 1984; Scaler Scott et al., 2014). It is important to note that because some of the diagnoses such as autism, Tourette syndrome, and anxiety often don't occur as early as preschool years, one can only ascertain in these "no other diagnosis" cases that there was no other diagnosis at the time of the stuttering evaluation. For the purposes of this book, references to atypical disfluencies will include:

- WFDs, including repetitions of final sounds or syllables
  - I went to the game-m last night(pause)ight.

  - I was glad that my team-eam won.

  The first sentence example includes a final sound repetition (game-m) and a final syllable repetition (night-ight). Note that in the example of the word "night," there is a pause before the syllable repetition, but in the second sentence example, where there is a WFD on the word "team," there is no pause. These different examples are used to make clear to the reader that each of these types of WFDs (with and without pauses before them) have been noted to occur in speech.

- Word-final repetitions with insertions
  - I don't know my way-hay home.

  Note that in the example, /h/ is inserted. This disfluency will be characterized as a WFD, because the entire word was spoken before the ending was added. Without the insertion of /h/, "way-ay" would be categorized as a word-final repetition. With the insertion of /h/, the only change is that the WFD now contains an insertion.

- Mid-word insertions
  - My tea-he-he-heacher is very nice.

  In this example, mid-word insertions are considered atypical disfluencies, as they are not commonly observed in stuttering. However, it is difficult to ascertain whether this is different from stuttering or if a client may be inserting a sound while they are struggling to move forward in a word, as in stuttering. The insertion of /h/ could be related to the client trying to take a breath during a stuttering block. Ways to analyze individual client patterns to distinguish atypical disfluencies from moments of stuttering will be discussed in the section on differential diagnosis.

Word-medial repetitions and prolongations will not be considered atypical disfluencies. Although they occur less frequently than stuttering on initial sounds or syllables, they have been documented to occur in this position in stuttered speech (Natke, Sandrieser, Van Ark, Pietrowsky, & Kalveram, 2004). Many clinicians may have observed their clients stuttering in the medial position of a multisyllabic word. Additionally, these were treated with traditional stuttering treatment methods in the Osborne

(2004) study and will be handled as such in the treatment section of this book. On the other hand, the WFDs outlined earlier will be treated with less traditional methods than those typically used for stuttering. The reason for this distinction in treatment is described in the treatment section of this chapter.

It is important to note that defining these types of disfluencies is currently in its infancy and that more research is needed. To date, however, these are the types of disfluencies that have been identified by clinicians and in research studies. For the most part, it has been documented that clients with atypical disfluencies present as unaware of their condition. However, documentation is beginning to emerge of cognitive components to this disorder, including misperception of how a child may have started using WFDs (Scaler Scott et al., 2014). It is likely safe to say that just as affective and cognitive components to cluttering have been recently identified in the literature, so might these components emerge among some people with atypical disfluencies.

## Excessive Non–Stuttering-Like Disfluencies That Are not Cluttering

Because this book is dealing with clients with concomitant disorders, there are cases where clients will present with excessive NSLDs—revisions of thought, interjections, and repetitions of phrases and/or words without tension (Ambrose & Yairi, 1999; Yairi & Ambrose, 1992)—but no breakdown in overall speech intelligibility. In these cases, the excessive NSLDs are likely due to difficulties with language retrieval and formulation issues. A client may present with stuttering and/or atypical disfluency and excessive NSLDs due to an accompanying language disorder. Therefore, it is worth mentioning in our definitions that these types of disfluencies would be related to language disorders and treated as such. More extensive coverage of differential diagnosis between cluttering and language-based disfluency will be covered later in this chapter.

# CURRENT STATE OF THE RESEARCH

## Stuttering

Although an exhaustive review of the literature is beyond the scope of this book, some of the most recent updates in stuttering research bear mentioning, as they may inform clinical decision making in evaluation and treatment.

Stuttering is considered multifactorial in its etiology, and several theories attempt to explain why a client may stutter. These include explanations that are based on differences in brain structure (Chang, Erickson, Ambrose, Hasegawa-Johnson, & Ludlow, 2008; De Nil, Kroll, Lafaille, & Houle, 2003), brain function (Braun et al., 1997; Chang, Kenney, Loucks, & Ludlow, 2009; De Nil, Beal, Lafaille, Kroll, Crawley, & Gracco, 2008; Fox et al., 1996; Fox et al., 2000; Lu et al., 2010), genetic links (see Yairi & Ambrose, 2013, for review), or difficulties with linguistic encoding tasks (Bernstein, 1981, Bernstein Ratner, 1997; Bloodstein, 2002, 2006; Karniol, 1995; Kolk & Postma, 1997; Packman, Onslow, Richard, & van Doorn, 1996; Perkins, Kent, & Curlee, 1991; Postma & Kolk, 1993). Differences in structure and function of the brain have been found in adults (Braun et al., 1997; Brown, Ingham, Ingham, Laird, & Fox, 2005; Chang et al., 2009; De Nil et al., 2003; De Nil et al., 2008; Fox et al., 1996; Fox et al., 2000; Lu et al., 2010; Wu et al., 1997) and children (Chang et al., 2008; Usler & Weber-Fox, 2015) who stutter, but findings have varied between studies. None have been shown to account for stuttering in all cases. The multifactorial theory of stuttering (Smith,1990a, 1990b; Smith & Kelly, 1997) is likely the most accepted theory among practicing clinicians (Smith, 1990a, 1990b; Smith & Kelly, 1997). This theory identifies that stuttering may be caused by a mix of factors, including neurological, genetic, and environmental. No one factor is thought to cause stuttering alone, but the three factors are thought to combine in different proportions in different clients. That is, whereas one client may have genetic and neurological factors that contribute to their stuttering, another may have all three factors. One client may have a majority of genetic factors, whereas another may have a majority of neurological factors. Many clients, because of genetic linkages within the family, are thought to have a predisposition to stuttering. Although the interaction of variables is complex, and genetic predisposition does not always equate to the development of stuttering (Yairi, Ambrose, & Cox, 1996), this genetic predisposition may triggers the stuttering at some point in the client's life. Although the stuttering may be triggered by a specific stressful event (e.g., a move, birth of a sibling, reading aloud in school), the combination of the predisposition, differences in neurology, and the stressful event at just the right timing is thought to trigger the stuttering rather than the specific stressful event alone. Following the logic of the theory of predisposition, even if this stressful event had never occurred, the stuttering may have emerged in response to another stressful event, as it was "predetermined" (by wiring and genetic makeup) to do so. This can be likened to recent findings in cancer research (Esteller, 2011), which indicate that although a patient may have a genetic link to a certain type of cancer, that person will need the right combination of factors to serve as the switch to turn that gene on (Esteller, 2011). This research is important for practicing clinicians to share with parents of children who stutter, as many parents will come looking for "the cause." Questions about cause are difficult to answer, and without this research support, parents may tend to blame themselves for the evolution of stuttering in their child ("I should have taken him for therapy sooner," "We never should have moved," "We never should have put her in that new school"). Parents and loved ones relate anxiety to stuttering because they see increased stuttering when their loved one appears anxious or upset. But it is important for family members to know that although anxiety may make stuttering worse, and although it has been found to sometimes present as a coexisting issue in stuttering, there is no evidence to show that anxiety is a sole cause of stuttering (see Bloodstein & Bernstein Ratner, 2008, for review). Table 2-2 shows myths associated with stuttering, their potential origin, what the current research shows about stuttering, and how this information applies clinically.

## Cluttering

As mentioned, the LCD definition of cluttering reflects several new updates in cluttering research. First, the reader should note that the mandatory criteria for a diagnosis of cluttering is perceived rapid or irregular rate of speech. Perceived is an important term to note. In the past, researchers and clinicians believed that a person with cluttering must always speak at a rate that is faster than average. Generally, a person with cluttering or suspected cluttering does sound fast to the listener. However, in prior research, the actual rate of speech in those with cluttering was not always specifically measured. Updated research (Raphael, Bakker, Myers, & St. Louis, 2010) has shown that speaking rate in cluttering is not always faster than average. Raphael et al. (2010) consider that the perception of rapid rate may be caused by the over-coarticulated syllables and/or an overall irregular rate. In some cases, the client with cluttering might pause less than the average speaker, making the perception of their rate faster than average, but not the actual rate (Scaler Scott et al., 2013). The theory in cluttering (Bakker, Myers, Raphael, & St. Louis, 2011; Myers, 1992) that is currently espoused is that the speaker is speaking at a rate that is too fast for their system to handle, thereby resulting in at least one of the cluttering symptoms in the LCD definition. The way to handle this perceived rapid and/or irregular rate will be discussed in detail in the sections on evaluation and differential diagnosis.

| TABLE 2-2 | | | |
|---|---|---|---|
| **Stuttering Myths, Potential Origins, Current Research, Clinical Implications** | | | |
| *STUTTERING MYTH* | *POSSIBLE ORIGIN* | *CURRENT RESEARCH* | *CLINICAL IMPLICATION* |
| Stuttering can be caused by parents. | Diagnosogenic theory (Johnson, 1955). Concept that stuttering begins by parents labeling a child's hesitations as stuttering. | Multifactorial theory (Smith, 1990a, 1990b; Smith & Kelly, 1997): Stuttering is caused by a mix of neurological, genetic, and environmental factors. These factors present themselves differently in different individuals who stutter. | Parents/caregivers are not at fault; if one stressor didn't exist, another likely would have triggered their child's stuttering. |
| Stuttering is caused by anxiety. | Appearance that stuttering gets worse when someone is stressed or anxious | Stuttering and anxiety may coexist; no evidence to support anxiety as sole cause of stuttering (Bloodstein & Bernstein Ratner, 2008). | Telling someone to "relax" or "calm down" is not helpful advice for stuttering. |

It was mentioned earlier that although it is not part of the LCD definition of cluttering, affective and cognitive components do exist and should be considered when evaluating someone with cluttering. In the past it was thought that those with cluttering had limited to no awareness of their communication disorder. Research has since revealed that just as in stuttering, some with cluttering have experienced negative reactions from others, have been underemployed due to their communication disorder, and have been engaged in avoidance behaviors because of their cluttering (Scaler Scott & St. Louis, 2011).

It is important to consider the topic of cluttering awareness from a new perspective. As previously described, cluttering is a disorder that, until recently, was relatively confusing and/or unknown among professionals and the public alike. Each time I speak at a workshop about diagnosing cluttering, at least one clinician reports that they feel that due to prior confusion over the cluttering definition, they may have misdiagnosed clients who were cluttering as stuttering. As awareness and education are increasing, improvements are noted, yet misdiagnoses still continue (Scaler Scott & St.

*...although anxiety may make stuttering worse...there is no evidence to show that anxiety is a sole cause of stuttering (see Bloodstein & Bernstein Ratner, 2008, for review).*

Louis, 2011). Among the public, it is likely still safe to say that although the average layperson may know that something is amiss in a speaker's communication skills, they would be unable to give a name to the communication disorder. It is one thing to be unaware that there is any problem whatsoever, and another to be aware there is a problem but to not have the correct terminology to link to the disorder. Reports from adults who clutter, including adults who were interviewed independently of each other, indicate that as a child, people would make vague remarks about improving their communication skills (Dewey, 2005; Scaler Scott & St. Louis, 2011). These adults with cluttering also reported being aware of confused looks from others. Therefore, they were aware that others couldn't understand them, but couldn't understand why. That is, they were aware of the existence of cluttering even when they couldn't give a name to it.

Those who clutter may be aware of their cluttering in general, but unaware in the moment the symptoms occur (Van Zaalen, Wijnen, & Dejonckere, 2011a). This is no different from someone who stutters not being acutely aware of every repetition, or a speaker without a fluency disorder being unaware of how frequently they use the filler word "um." Because previous literature mentioned a lack of awareness among those who clutter, before the LCD definition, many clinicians informally adopted the lack of awareness as a way of differentiating stuttering from cluttering. Given the latest research findings on awareness, using awareness as a criteria for differential diagnosis of stuttering from cluttering is no longer appropriate.

Another possibility related to lack of awareness is lack of readiness to accept the communication disorder. Several people with cluttering have reported that in their teen years, they often defended their cluttering as being in the ear of their listener rather than an actual problem. But when reflecting back on those years, these adults stated that they were not yet ready to take responsibility for their communication disorder (Scaler Scott & St. Louis, 2011). This lack of readiness is again different from a lack of awareness in general. As we will discuss in detail in the differential diagnosis section, awareness should be evaluated on a case-by-case basis.

Before the LCD definition of cluttering was put forward, many references to diagnosing cluttering referred to accompanying difficulties with language. The authors of the LCD definition acknowledge the fact that some with cluttering may also have accompanying language disorders (St. Louis & Schulte, 2011). But current research has taught us that all people with cluttering do not have an accompanying language disorder. Therefore, language-related symptoms are not part of the LCD of what we hear as clinicians when we listen to someone who clutters. Difficulties with verbal organization have recently been identified in cluttering, in various speaking contexts (Bretherton-Furness & Ward, 2012), and during speech tasks under functional magnetic resonance imaging (Ward, Connally, Pliatsikas, & Bretherton-Furness, 2015). However, differences in the language portions of the brain have not yet been identified (Ward et al., 2015). It is currently debated whether the differences are based on the organization of language rather than on a language disorder itself. It remains to be seen as to whether difficulty organizing thoughts is later added to the LCD definition of cluttering. For now, we consider that if clients meet the LCD definition criteria, they are cluttering. Anything seen in addition to these symptoms is viewed as a concomitant disorder.

*...awareness should be evaluated on a case-by-case basis.*

One final misconception that I have observed clinically is the concept that whereas stuttering may be situationally based, cluttering occurs each time a speaker attempts to communicate. It is difficult to trace the origins of this thinking, but I hypothesize that perhaps when cluttering was thought of as a "syndrome," many expected its features to be constant rather than intermittent, as one might expect in someone with Down syndrome. What has long been documented in the literature is that those with cluttering often "normalize" when they are aware they are being recorded. This is theorized to be because as client awareness of the recording increases, so does self-monitoring, which causes them to speak at a rate that is better for their system to handle. Continuing with this line of thinking, one should assume that when they are aware they are being evaluated, some clients may show decreased symptoms. This does not necessarily exclude the client from a diagnosis of cluttering. Additionally, Ward et al. (2015) describe the idea of "cluttering spectrum behavior," which states that some who clutter may do so only in specific situations, such as when giving a work presentation. The LCD definition reflects the idea that those with cluttering do not need to clutter a majority of the time to receive a diagnosis. Table 2-3 displays cluttering myths, research updates, and clinical implications.

| TABLE 2-3 | | | |
|---|---|---|---|
| **Cluttering Myths, Potential Origins, Current Research, Clinical Implications** | | | |
| *CLUTTERING MYTH* | *POSSIBLE ORIGIN* | *CURRENT RESEARCH* | *CLINICAL IMPLICATION* |
| Those who clutter speak faster than average. | Sounding faster than average to the listener | Rate is not always faster than average (St. Louis & Schulte, 2011); speaker is speaking at a rate that is too fast for their system to handle (Bakker et al., 2011; Myers, 1992); perception of rapid rate may be caused by the over-coarticulated syllables and/or an overall irregular rate (Raphael et al., 2010). | Perceived rapid rate rather than measured rapid rate is sufficient for a diagnosis |
| Those who clutter lack awareness of their communication disorder. | Confusion about true lack of awareness vs. knowledge of the correct terminology to describe their symptoms | Those who clutter may be aware of the disorder but not aware in the moment it is occurring (Van Zaalen et al., 2011a). | Lack of awareness will vary by individual and should be individually evaluated. |
| Those who clutter do not experience affective and cognitive components. | May be related to misconception that all with cluttering are unaware of their symptoms | Affective and cognitive components are documented in recent interviews with adults with cluttering (Scaler Scott & St. Louis, 2011). | Evaluate for affective and cognitive components to determine the overall impact of the disorder on each client. |
| Those who clutter must do so in a majority of speaking situations to be diagnosed with cluttering. | Possibly came from idea that cluttering was described as an overall "syndrome" | LCD definition states that clear instances of cluttering even a minority of the time are sufficient for diagnosis (St. Louis & Schulte, 2011). | Evaluate client in multiple contexts, including contexts reported by client and/or significant others to trigger symptoms. |

## *Atypical Disfluencies*

The latest research reflects the fact that there is still debate about 1) whether atypical disfluencies are actually a form of stuttering or something else and 2) what the best treatment strategies may be regarding atypical disfluencies. The majority of research on this topic until present has documented that these disfluencies exist and in what populations they have been identified. The disfluencies have been identified in those with neurological differences (Doi et al., 2003; Lebrun & Leleux, 1985; Van Borsel, Van Coster, & Van Lierd, 1996) but also in those with no other known disorder (Camarata, 1989; McAllister & Kingston, 2005; Mowrer, 1987; Rudmin, 1984). Some researchers have hypothesized what might underlie such disfluencies. Some of the hypotheses espoused include a type of disfluency on the stuttering continuum with difficulty terminating the final syllable of a word (just as someone who stutters often has difficulty initiating the first syllable of a word; Van Borsel, Geirnaert, & Van Coster, 2005; Cosyns et al., 2010), cognitive processing difficulties (McAllister & Kingston, 2005), perseveration (Sisskin & Wasilus, 2014), and attempts to regulate phonological production (Camarata, 1989; Mowrer, 1984; Rudmin, 1984; Stansfield, 1995). Despite a growing but still small body of literature related to atypical disfluencies, more and more clinicians are asking what the take-away clinical recommendation is for these disfluencies. Given that more research is needed, experts are recommending that clinicians engage in their own hypothesis testing with each individual client to determine what function the atypical disfluencies may serve (Scaler Scott & Sisskin, 2007). For example, speakers without fluency disorders often uses interjections such as "um" and "uh" to hold the floor while trying to retrieve a word or organize thoughts (Clark & Fox Tree, 2002). Clinicians are advised to study each client and determine if the atypical disfluency might be serving such a purpose for them. If it is, for example, serving a purpose of the client needing more time to formulate a thought, then the clinician might address language formulation in their session. I have found some clinical success with helping clients in this area, as well as some other areas, based upon results of extensive testing on a small sample of school-aged children with atypical disfluencies (Sutkowski, Tokach, & Scaler Scott, 2015). How to evaluate and treat this difficulty will be discussed more in the relevant evaluation and treatment sections of this book.

One of the hypotheses that my research team continues to explore is that of working memory. This hypothesis is related to the idea that in conversation or monologue contexts, where individuals tend to exhibit the greatest number of disfluencies, working memory is required. This concept has been supported by the idea that when people with atypical disfluencies are interrupted, thus taxing their working memory, their WFDs tend to increase (Scaler Scott et al., 2013). Anecdotally, several of my clients with WFDs have reported that they do not like interruptions from others when they are speaking, as they are afraid they will forget what they are going to say. When interruptions are placed in the context of a game, the speakers showed increased WFDs upon being interrupted. Publication of results of increased WFDs during interruptions is in process, but given the small sample size, replication will be required before generalizing findings. Clinically, I have found that teaching clients to use visualization strategies to strengthen working memory has shown some reduction in WFDs (Scaler Scott et al., 2014).

# ASSESSMENT AND DIFFERENTIAL DIAGNOSIS

## *Fluency Evaluation in General*

We will begin with a discussion of how to conduct an overall fluency evaluation. By preparing for a fluency evaluation in general, the clinician will be setting themselves up for the most comprehensive means of differential diagnosis. It is important to consider that due to lack of awareness among the general public regarding cluttering, atypical disfluency, and covert stuttering, a client who is initially referred for stuttering may be found to only outwardly exhibit NSLDs. For this reason, starting with a general fluency evaluation and using the methods that follow for differential diagnosis will allow the clinician to gain the best understanding of their client's needs overall.

Speaking samples in a variety of contexts are most important to gather for a fluency evaluation. These contexts should include (at minimum) reading, conversation, and monologue. Aiming for a 5-minute sample during conversation and monologue will help ensure that you have enough words/syllables to analyze. Depending upon circumstances, the clinician may also want to ask for a home speech sample to analyze, or perhaps a speech sample from a work presentation in the case of the adult client. In general, if it is felt by the client or significant other(s) that relevant fluency characteristics may not be observed in the evaluation session, obtaining samples from whatever the relevant contexts are should be encouraged.

Conducting a disfluency analysis on each of these samples will provide a broad context of the types of disfluencies the client exhibits. The clinician must either transcribe each speaking sample word for word and code the disfluencies, or listen to each sample and code (with a quick symbol such as a dot) each word or syllable and type of disfluency (with relevant symbols) as they are heard. It is recommended that clinicians code moments of the following categories to help in later differential diagnosis: 1) SLDs; 2) NSLDs; 3) atypical disfluencies; 4) moments of atypical pausing; and 5) moments of over-coarticulation. It is important to note that "moments of" refer to "instances of." That is, if a client exhibits a part-word repetition with either 3 repetitions of a syllable (e.g., li-li-li-like) or 10 repetitions of a syllable (e.g., li-li-li-li-li-li-li-li-li-li-like), this would in both cases count as one moment of a syllable repetition. This would also apply to repetitions at the end of a word (e.g., like-ike) for a WFD. Likewise, if a client were to repeat a whole word one time or six times, that repetition would be one moment of whole word repetition (Yaruss, 1998). Sample transcripts highlighting each type of disfluency for reading, conversation, and monologue are located in Appendices B, C, and D. Two types of transcripts are presented to illustrate different options for the clinician. It is important to note that although this practice can be quite time consuming, if done well for the evaluation, it often helps the clinician to sort out any confusion in differential diagnosis. If saving time is of essence, coding the longest sample of connected speech, such as monologue, will provide the greatest amount of information. Monologue has been found to reveal the most instances of over-coarticulated in school-aged children who clutter (Scaler Scott, Kidron, & Lozier, 2012).

After all words are transcribed and coded, the clinician should do a word count of all meaningful words in the transcript. Meaningful words are those that add to the content of the passage (Yaruss, 1998). Therefore, repetitions of whole words or interjections would not count as meaningful words. Once the number of meaningful words is calculated, the clinician can then count all the instances of the categories coded earlier and divide each by the number of meaningful words to obtain the percentage of each type of disfluency. One note of caution is that when the clinician is calculating categories such as NSLDs, all that is included in the numerator must be in the denominator. So, for example, even though interjections are not considered meaningful words, we cannot calculate the percentage of interjections if they are not included in the denominator. Therefore, those types of words initially excluded may be included depending upon the type of disfluency one is calculating. Within each larger category, instances of specific types of disfluencies can also be calculated. For example, the clinician should calculate the percentage of total SLDs that are blocks, repetitions, or prolongations; the percentage of total NSLDs that are interjections, revisions, whole word, or phrase repetitions; and the percentage of atypical disfluencies that occur with or without a pause (reasons for considering this final aspect will be described in relevant treatment sections throughout this book).

Analyzing this sample of connected speech will give the clinician a clear example of whether to look further into stuttering, cluttering, and/or atypical disfluencies. In terms of stuttering, 3% or greater syllables stuttered (Conture, 2001) is the initial criterion to achieve this diagnosis. Keep in mind that the percentage of overt behaviors may be less in someone who is hiding their stuttering (i.e., covert stutterer) and that a smaller percentage is not necessarily grounds for determining whether a person stutters until all factors are examined. The presence of secondary behaviors should also be factored into the diagnosis of stuttering, although their presence is not mandatory for a diagnosis. There are conflicting findings regarding the frequency of NSLDs in typical adult speakers (see Schleef, 2005, for review). In an analysis of the type of filler words used by academic instructors and students, Schleef (2005) found that college students (high of 20 per 1,000 words) tended to produce more fillers as compared to instructors (high of 6 per 1,000 words), and females tended to produce more fillers as compared with males.

In terms of cluttering, in addition to transcribing the sample, the clinician should listen to the sample(s) to gain an impression as to whether the rate sounds rapid or irregular. A measure of speech rate can be taken, but because the LCD definition focuses on perceived rapid or irregular rate, measuring speech rate is not a key deciding factor. Furthermore, the client's speech may be perceived as rapid (sufficient for meeting the mandatory criterion of cluttering) but not measure at a higher-than-average rate. Recall that the client does not need to exhibit this rapid or irregular rate in all situations. Therefore, even if a specific sample does not include perceived rapid or irregular rate, cluttering cannot be completely ruled out until all speaking contexts are examined. If it is determined that the client does exhibit rapid or irregular rate in specific contexts, the next three criteria for a diagnosis of cluttering should be examined in the transcripts of those context(s). That is, the transcript should be examined for excessive NSLDs, moments of over-coarticulation, and/or moments of atypical pausing.

Regarding the NSLDs, it should be kept in mind that the LCD definition does not indicate a minimum percentage to meet the criteria for cluttering. The definition simply specifies "excessive." This is because the research does not yet have a specific percentage that would serve as a baseline for diagnosis. In the meantime, the clinician is encouraged to consider something as "excessive" when it has a negative functional impact upon a client's ability to communicate efficiently and effectively. For example, if the client were to exhibit so many revisions and/or interjections that it was difficult to either ascertain or follow their message, this would be determined to be clinically relevant, as it has negative functional impact upon a client's communication. Many times reading the transcript will help demonstrate this; however, the clinician may feel that listening to the sample also allows for a better decision on communication effectiveness. Should the clinician require numerical support (for reimbursement purposes or for qualifying for services), it may be helpful to document the percentage of NSLDs vs. SLDs. Many times the disparity between a very low percentage of SLDs as compared to a higher number of NSLDs is a useful way to show how excessive NSLDs interfere with effective communication. This may not apply, however, if the client both stutters and clutters, as both percentages may be high, or the SLDs may be higher. When needing to advocate for cluttering intervention for a client, I have found that the most telling way to illustrate this to the reader is to provide a sample of the transcript containing excessive disfluencies in the written evaluation report. This helps paint a picture of the negative impact of excessive NSLDs on a client's communication effectiveness that someone outside the field of speech-language pathology (such as a principal, parent, or teacher) can understand.

*In order to receive a diagnosis of cluttering, a client will need to exhibit clear instances of rapid or irregular rate, as well as exhibit at least one of the three criteria outlined in the LCD definition.*

For moments of over-coarticulated, there is also no percentage established as a criterion. The clinician is again asked to determine the overall negative impact of these instances on the client's intelligibility—that is, asking whether the client exhibits so many moments of over-coarticulated that it is difficult to understand what they are saying. Painting a picture by providing a sample of their transcript in written documentation is often helpful to illustrate this concept. Please refer to Appendix A for sample report excerpts.

In terms of atypical pausing, it will be useful to look at the transcript and mark areas where the client paused. The clinician can then mark areas where pauses are expected. Marking both expected and actual pauses will help to illustrate 1) how often the client is pausing (i.e., are the sentences longer than you would expect with little pausing?) and 2) how often pausing occurs in unexpected places. It is important to note that it is unlikely that 100% of a person's cluttering-related pauses occur in unexpected places. Also, the clinician will want to listen to the speech sample(s) to determine whether the client's speech sounds "jerky" or "spurty" in terms of rhythm. This is often due to placement of pauses.

Remember: In order to receive a diagnosis of cluttering, a client will need to exhibit clear instances of rapid or irregular rate, as well as exhibit at least one of the three criteria outlined in the LCD definition.

Examples of analyzed transcripts, including symptoms of cluttering, are included in Appendices B, C, and D.

| TABLE 2-4 | | |
| --- | --- | --- |
| **Examples of Available Tools for Assessing Affective and Cognitive Components of Fluency Disorders** | | |
| *NAME OF TOOL* | *AUTHOR(S)/(PUBLISHERS)* | *POPULATIONS AND AGES* |
| Overall Assessment of the Speaker's Experience of Stuttering | Yaruss, Quesal, Coleman (Stuttering Therapy Resources, 2006) | Versions available for children (7 to 12), teens (13 to 17), and adults; examines knowledge and feelings about stuttering, response toward stuttering; overall impact score available; norm referenced |
| What's True for You? from *The School-Aged Child who Stutters: Working Effectively with Attitudes and Emotions* | Chmela & Reardon (Stuttering Foundation of America, 2001) | Informal checklist for school-aged children (begins at age 9). |
| Wright and Ayre Stuttering Self-Rating Profile (WASSP) | Wright & Ayre (Speechmark, 2006) | Assesses thoughts and feelings about stuttering in adults |
| Behavior Assessment Battery for School-aged Children Who Stutter | Brutten & Vanryckeghem (Plural Publishing, 2006) | For children ages 6 through 15; provides three different checklists with normative data. Evaluates a child's 1) emotional reaction to speech disruption; 2) coping strategies for dealing with disfluency; and 3) general attitudes about speech (can be used with any type of disfluency, not specific to stuttering); norm referenced; includes KiddyCAT for preschool and kindergarten children. |
| KiddyCAT | Vanryckeghem & Brutten (Plural Publishing, 2006) | Assesses thoughts, feelings, reactions to stuttering in preschool and kindergarten children |

## *Atypical Disfluencies*

There are no diagnostic criteria for diagnosis of atypical disfluencies. The clinician would simply use the coded transcript to identify whether the client is exhibiting these patterns of disfluencies. Just as with cluttering, it is often helpful if the clinician includes several examples of atypical disfluencies in the evaluation report to identify functional impact (or lack thereof). Forthcoming research suggests a full assessment of language organization, formulation, and language memory may be warranted (Sutkowski, Tokach, & Scaler Scott, 2015) in clients with atypical disfluencies. This comprehensive assessment of skills is not necessary in order to identify the presence of atypical disfluencies, but will help to inform future treatment, as will be discussed.

As mentioned, the affective and cognitive components of fluency should be explored as well, regardless of the type of fluency disorder(s) a client presents with. These components can be explored via a checklist that examines communication attitudes in general, or one specific to stuttering (if stuttering is confirmed to be the only diagnosis present). Several checklists are described in Table 2-4. If the standard score offered by a formal questionnaire is not needed, the clinician can also interview the adult or child about feelings regarding their communication disorder, possible avoidances or "tricks" used, etc. It is important to note two things when conducting such an interview: 1) The clinician should ask all questions and record all answers in a nonjudgmental manner, regardless of the responses provided. For example, if a client indicates that they change their name to something different to avoid stuttering during introductions, the clinician should maintain a "neutral face" and record the response. The evaluation is not the time to educate a client why their coping strategy may not be the most effective.

For children, I find it particularly helpful to tell them that some people who stutter have figured out ways around their stuttering that they feel are helpful. I then follow this statement by asking, "So do you use anything like this?" Putting it out there that others may use "tricks" helps a child to see that we are not judging them for using the tricks. If a client feels judged about use of a coping strategy and feels the "right" answer is to say that they never, for example, avoid their stuttering, they then may provide this answer because they feel they are "supposed to." When the client answers in this manner, the clinician does not obtain a true picture of the client's status. Therefore, remaining as neutral and nonjudgmental as possible during the evaluation process is extremely important to gaining an accurate assessment.

*The affective and cognitive components of fluency should be explored, regardless of the type of fluency disorder(s) with which a client presents.*

There will be time during later therapy sessions, after trust and rapport are well established, to explore more effective solutions rather than avoidance of disfluency. 2) Simply because it is often the client's first time meeting the clinician, they may be apt to share less than they would once rapport has been built throughout therapy sessions. Therefore, it is important to keep in mind that not all answers may be obtained at the initial evaluation session. A good clinician is comfortable with the idea that not all answers are definitive, but a strong evaluation can provide a strong start from which hypotheses should be further explored in therapy.

It is important to note that because all three or some combination of the three fluency disorders may occur in the same client, all types of disfluencies and their potential interaction should be considered during the evaluation. Additionally, because many who exhibit cluttering and/or atypical disfluencies have been noted to present with co-occurring diagnoses, and because as many as 63% of children with stuttering may also present with concomitant disorders (Blood, Ridenour, Qualls, & Hammer, 2003), it is important to understand whatever fluency symptoms are identified in the context

*Because all three or some combination of the three fluency disorders may occur in the same client, all types of disfluencies and their potential interaction should be considered during the evaluation.*

of all presenting symptoms of the client. The section on differential diagnosis will help the clinician make judgments about whether a symptom is truly that of a specific fluency disorder or related to a co-occurring diagnosis. Additionally, this section will guide the clinician to think about how various fluency disorders may interact.

# DIFFERENTIAL DIAGNOSIS

The easiest way to discuss making a differential diagnosis is to focus on ruling out cluttering. This is because cluttering symptoms overlap with those of stuttering and other language disorders. Therefore, examining each potential cluttering symptom in turn allows for a thorough differential diagnosis. For each of the diagnostic criteria for cluttering, it is important to examine whether cluttering is the root cause of that symptom. For example, as shown later, excessive NSLDs may be rooted in cluttering, avoidance of stuttering, or a language disorder. We will take each potential cluttering symptom in turn to outline how to differentially diagnose cluttering from other disorders.

## Perceived Rapid and/or Irregular Rate

It is important to note here that use of a rapid or irregular rate is not seen in cluttering exclusively. Clients may use a rapid or irregular rate in other neurological disorders, like palilalia, or psychiatric disorders, such as schizophrenia (Andreasen & Grove, 1986). Additionally, clients who stutter sometimes may speed up in order to avoid a moment of stuttering. Speeding up will not always lead to cluttering symptoms. That is, the client may be a covert stutterer who uses increased rate to maintain fluency and/or to avoid moments of stuttering. If the client increases speed to avoid stuttering and this does not trigger symptoms of cluttering, then the client would only qualify for a diagnosis of covert stuttering. If the client increases speed to avoid stuttering and this does trigger symptoms of cluttering, then the client would qualify for a diagnosis of covert stuttering and cluttering. This would mean that as the client increased speed, they began speaking at a rate that was too fast for their system to handle, and this triggered cluttering symptoms. It does not mean that the client's avoidance of stuttering caused the cluttering, but rather the avoidance triggered the cluttering in someone who was already predisposed to clutter. Whether a rapid or irregular rate results in cluttering symptoms or not, it is important to understand the root cause of the client's increased rate. For example, if increased speed is related to avoidance of stuttering, then this avoidance needs to be dealt with in order to help the client make meaningful change. If the increased speed is related to a lack of self-regulation, then self-regulation will be the root issue targeted in therapy. We will discuss addressing the root issue further when we discuss treatment.

> *Whether a rapid or irregular rate results in cluttering symptoms or not, it is important to understand the root cause of the client's increased rate.*

## Excessive Non–Stuttering-Like Disfluencies

Although NSLDs may be the result of a client speaking at a rate that is faster than their system can handle, they also can be due to other communication disorders, such as difficulties with language formulation or word finding. If the clinician suspects this may be an issue, formal testing of language formulation, vocabulary, and/or word finding may be warranted. Those who stutter, clutter, and/or have atypical disfluencies may have accompanying language disorders. Therefore, it may be difficult at times to determine whether excessive revisions are related to difficulties with cluttering or language formulation. What is fairly consistent about cluttering is that when a client adjusts their rate to be more in line with a speed their system can keep up with, their cluttering symptoms tend to dissipate. Therefore, if trying to determine whether a client's excessive revisions are related to cluttering or to difficulties with formulation/retrieval, the clinician can 1) administer formal language tests and analyze results for quantitative and qualitative differences and 2) have the client adjust their rate while speaking in the same context (e.g., monologue, conversation) and note whether excessive NSLDs decrease or disappear. Keep in mind that clients can have difficulties with language formulation that only show up in qualitative patterns (rather than quantitative scores) on standardized tests. Be on the lookout for such qualitative patterns. If none of these qualitative patterns or quantitative scores are seen and adjusting rate results in decreased NSLDs, it is likely you are dealing with cluttering and not language formulation issues.

It also bears noting that if someone is trying to avoid or escape moments of stuttering, they may engage in use of excessive interjections to get started or continue what they are saying without stuttering. They also may be aware of an upcoming word upon which they feel they will stutter. If this happens, they may revise their thought once or several times to avoid that word or engage in word substituting, which may sound like a revision. Whether a client engages in avoidance behavior should be discussed in a nonjudgmental manner during the evaluation session. It is possible, however, that the client may not disclose their avoidance behaviors during the evaluation session. These and other covert aspects a client may be engaging in should be explored throughout the therapy process as rapport and trust continue to be established and built.

### Excessive Over-Coarticulation

As with the other symptoms of cluttering, the symptom of over-coarticulated may be the sign of other disorders. For example, a client with dysarthria might exhibit over-coarticulated. In these instances, having the client decrease their rate while talking and observing the difference can be invaluable. Upon decreasing the rate, the person with cluttering (without coexisting articulation and/or oral motor disorder) should exhibit clear, articulate, intelligible speech. If there are any concomitant articulation errors, such as a distorted /r/, they will remain, but syllables will no longer be over-coarticulated. By contrast, if someone with dysarthria slows down, their speech is likely to be more clear and intelligible than it previously was, but distortion of sounds will remain. I often give a formal articulation test to a client who I think may be cluttering as a standard part of the evaluation battery. Giving such a test allows me to 1) determine whether there are concomitant articulation errors and, if so, in what contexts and 2) demonstrate that the client can accurately produce sounds at the single-word level.

*In cluttering, remember that the difficulty is not related to correct articulation of specific sounds... the breakdown is related to speaking at a rate that is faster than the speaker's system can handle.*

In cluttering, remember that the difficulty is not related to correct articulation of specific sounds. What sounds are over-coarticulated can vary from one speaking context to the next. This is because the breakdown is related to speaking at a rate that is faster than the speaker's system can handle.

Demonstrating that articulation scores are normal helps to illustrate that cluttering is not an articulation disorder but a disorder related to rate that occurs in connected speech. If there is a concomitant articulation disorder, testing results can also highlight the fact that the errors are consistent (keeping in mind that there is a range of consistency with articulation and phonological disorders that varies between clients), whereas the sounds upon which over-coarticulated is produced are inconsistent from one word and from one speaking context to the next.

### Abnormal Pauses, Syllable Stress, and Speech Rhythm

To reiterate, this is not the atypical prosody noted in clients on the autism spectrum. A client with cluttering may have speech that sounds "jerky" or "spurty" because they frequently revise utterances (excessive NSLDs) and/or place pauses in places not expected grammatically. They may not use as many pauses in their everyday speech, and therefore may end up speaking too long on one breath and be forced to take a breath in places that are not expected grammatically. Another factor to consider when analyzing this variable is whether the client has difficulty with word finding and/or verbal formulation, causing them to pause in unexpected places to give themselves time to retrieve a word or thought. Conducting standardized testing of word retrieval skills will help determine the root cause of the atypical pauses so that the appropriate difficulty can be addressed in treatment (i.e., rate regulation vs. word retrieval skills). Finally, difficulties with motor planning due to apraxia of speech and that factor's possible contribution to atypical speech rhythm should be ruled out.

## Mid-Word Insertions Versus Stuttering Blocks

As mentioned earlier in the chapter, a client who says "my tea-he-he-he-heacher" may either be exhibiting a stuttering block or a mid-word insertion (atypical disfluency). At times clients use an /h/ as a means of trying to take a breath in response to a stuttering block. If the client 1) seems to have an overall pattern of stuttering blocks throughout the collected speech samples (regardless of any other fluency diagnoses) and 2) exhibits tension and struggle while attempting to produce a word, it is likely that their pattern is related to stuttering blocks. If the client 1) seems to have an overall pattern of disfluencies without tension throughout the collected speech samples and 2) exhibits no tension and struggle in the productions of "he" (as in during "tea-he-he-heacher"), it is likely that their pattern is related to atypical disfluency. I have found that most fluency clients do exhibit patterns, and once you look carefully for and identify these patterns, it is easier to reach a diagnosis.

# CASE EXAMPLE: DIFFERENTIAL DIAGNOSIS

## Background

Luke Hansen was a 6-year-old male who was brought to this clinician's attention due to difficulties with stuttering. Luke's mother, Mrs. Hansen, described Luke's stuttering as sounds getting stuck, accompanied by facial tension and beginning signs of avoidance, such as saying, "Forget it" and abandoning his utterance. Mr. and Mrs. Hansen indicated that Luke had received early intervention services as a preschooler, including speech-language therapy for a mild language delay and occupational therapy for sensory integration issues (sensory seeker). They further reported that Luke was discharged from services at age 4 due to language development being within normal limits and sensory integration symptoms being managed by a home sensory diet (i.e., trampoline, wheelbarrow walking, involvement in sports activities). The Hansens noted that early on, attention deficit hyperactivity disorder had been questioned but had been ruled out, as symptoms were thought to be related to sensory integration issues rather than attention. Upon initial consultation, the Hansens described Luke as like "peeling an onion" in that each year they felt a new layer of difficulty in some area of development emerged. They considered the stuttering just another layer.

Luke presented as a happy child who actively engaged the clinician in conversation. He was active and required frequent verbal redirection to his seat, to which he responded well. Stuttering was characterized by initial part-word repetitions and silent blocks of three seconds or less. When asked about his "bumpy speech," Luke indicated that he was aware and that it made him feel "sad." He denied changing words to help with fluency, and his parents confirmed that they had not observed any word avoidance. The clinician watched carefully for examples of word avoidance during the initial evaluation (e.g., blocking on a word and revising to another word, "I play outside on my tram—bouncy thing"), and none were observed. In a conversation with the Hansens where Luke was not present, the clinician explained how to watch for similar instances of word avoidance. I often have parents put such a plan of watching for avoidance into place because if a parent is not actively monitoring for signs of word substitution, they may not be aware substitution is occurring. Once it is pointed out to them exactly what to look for, parents may note more instances after the evaluation, which would inform future treatment. This is very often true of atypical disfluencies. That is, many parents are unaware they are occurring, but become acutely aware once the disfluencies are pointed out to them.

## Evaluation Procedures and Results

Luke was evaluated the summer before his first-grade year and was already a voracious and proficient reader. For the evaluation, conversation, monologue, and reading samples were recorded. Analysis of these samples revealed 6% stuttering-like fluencies, characterized by repetitions of single-syllable whole words of up to four repetitions (repetitions are also known as "iterations") and mild blocks of 3 seconds or less. Facial tension was observed during blocks. Analysis also revealed 5% NSLDs characterized by revisions, phrase repetitions, and interjections (um, uh, like). Intelligibility was good in known and unknown contexts, and the Hansens had no concerns with intelligibility of speech in daily communication exchanges. Fluency analysis revealed 0% moments of over-coarticulated and 0% atypical pauses (not counted during this analysis were pauses due to stuttering blocks, as these are part of stuttering and not cluttering). Instances of word finding were noted during conversation and play (i.e., "The fish has big … like those things on a lady's mouth"). To rule out word finding difficulties, the Test of Word Finding (German, 2015) was administered. Luke received a standard score of 93 on this test, indicating skills within the low-average range of performance. The Hansens did report similar instances of word finding in Luke's daily conversational speech. Articulation errors included substitution of /f/ for voiceless "th" and /d/ for voiced "th," both of which were considered within normal limits for his age. Luke's fluency analysis also revealed 0% atypical disfluencies. Because these disfluencies might not occur in all contexts, they were modeled for the Hansens, who denied having heard any instances of this type of disfluency. They were instructed to monitor for the appearance of any atypical disfluencies.

## Conclusions

Initial evaluation revealed a child with SLDs characterized by behavioral and affective components (i.e., feeling "sad" about his stuttering). No evidence of atypical disfluencies or cluttering was revealed. Word finding difficulties were noted. Although Luke and the Hansens both denied word switching, this pattern would continue to be monitored in treatment to ensure that word finding was truly word finding and not a stuttering avoidance behavior.

## Clinical Update: Peeling the Next Layer of the Onion

Two years after initiating stuttering treatment, Luke was being seen by the clinician (at parent request) three times a year to monitor fluency. It was about this time that the Hansens emerged with new concerns. They noted that they and others reported increased rate of speech and difficulty understanding what Luke was saying. The clinician obtained new fluency samples in the context of reading, monologue, and conversation. Analysis revealed 2% SLDs characterized by single-syllable whole word repetitions with mild tension and 5% NSLDs characterized by revisions, fillers, and phrase repetitions. Moments of over-coarticulated made up 10% of the words in the sample. Atypical disfluencies and atypical pauses were not evidenced during this sample. The Hansens confirmed that Luke was not exhibiting any new signs except for the rapid and over-coarticulated speech. From ongoing observation, Luke did not appear to be developing any negative communication attitudes. However, given Luke's history of stuttering, it was important to rule out possible emerging patterns of avoidance. That is to say, Luke might now be increasing his rate of speech to avoid moments of stuttering. Patterns of avoidance in chronic stuttering have been noted to develop in children over time, especially as the child becomes older and more aware of their stuttering (Guitar, 1998). Therefore, this was important to rule out. Parents were advised to monitor for signs of word or communication avoidance and to remind Luke that if he stuttered sometimes, it was still okay and that most important to them was hearing his message.

Overall, it appeared that Luke's stuttering remained status quo and that cluttering was emerging. Nonetheless, as a safeguard, the Hansens were instructed to keep reiterating (in action and in words) that they wanted first and foremost to hear what Luke had to say, whether or not he stuttered. I had witnessed the Hansens putting this idea into place over the years, but wanted to make sure that as Luke might be changing his thinking about whether or not it is okay to stutter (this can happen independently of what others tell the child), the Hansens were not wavering from their original stance. I found it to be the case that they remained solid in their acceptance and response to Luke's stuttering and that Luke did not seem to be experiencing any negative feelings or thoughts regarding his stuttering. As previously mentioned, this was important to figure out because if Luke had been speeding up to avoid stuttering, although this would not be the root cause of his new cluttering behavior, the stuttering avoidance would be the first problem to be addressed. That is, if you tell someone to increase pausing to decrease their rate (and to help cluttering), if they are still afraid of stuttering, they will have a hard time putting this strategy into practice until the avoidance and fear are addressed. Because Luke did not present with avoidance, it appeared that Luke perhaps always had the propensity to clutter and was just beginning to do so as his language was becoming more complex and lengthy. Therefore, work on rate regulation was in order. Treatment strategies for rate regulation in cluttering will be discussed in later chapters. What follows are three checklists the clinician can use and questions to guide in differential diagnosis.

# ASSESSMENT CHECKLIST: STUTTERING

☐ Concomitant disorders?

☐ Types of samples obtained:
    ☐ Reading
    ☐ Conversation
    ☐ Monologue
    ☐ Picture description
    ☐ Story retell
    ☐ Other

☐ Percentage of syllables stuttered:

☐ Types and percentages of SLDs:
    ☐ Part-word repetitions:
    ☐ Whole word repetitions:
    ☐ Prolongations:
    ☐ Blocks:

☐ Secondary behaviors:

☐ Affective components?

☐ Cognitive components?

☐ Avoidance and other covert behaviors?

# ASSESSMENT CHECKLIST: CLUTTERING

☐ Percentage of NSLDs:


☐ Types and percentages of NSLDs:
    ☐ Phrase repetitions:
    ☐ Revisions:
    ☐ Interjections:


☐ Percentage of words over-coarticulated:


☐ Percentage of atypical pauses:


☐ Affective components?


☐ Cognitive components?


☐ Communication avoidance?

# ASSESSMENT CHECKLIST: ATYPICAL DISFLUENCIES

☐ Types and percentages:

    ☐ Word-final syllable repetitions with pause:

    ☐ Word-final syllable repetitions without pause:

    ☐ Word-final sound repetitions with pause:

    ☐ Word-final sound repetitions without pause:

    ☐ Word-final prolongations:

☐ Mid-word insertions (percentage):

    ☐ Is there tension or no tension with the insertions?

    ☐ Is there a pattern of stuttering blocks?

☐ Affective components?

☐ Cognitive components?

☐ Communication avoidance?

# QUESTIONS TO ASK FOR DIFFERENTIAL DIAGNOSIS

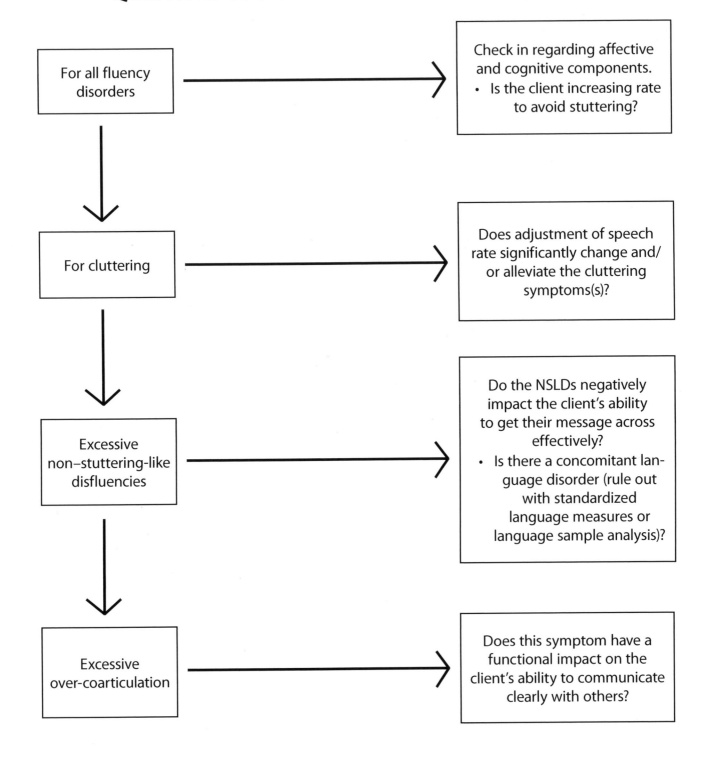

# APPENDIX A: EXAMPLE OF CLUTTERING EVALUATION REPORT OUTLINING WHETHER CRITERIA ARE MET FOR DIAGNOSIS

## Criterion #1: Mandatory for Diagnosis of Cluttering

Cluttering is a fluency disorder characterized by a rate that is perceived to be abnormally rapid, irregular, or both for the speaker (although measured syllable rates may not exceed normal limits; St. Louis & Schulte, 2011).

In conversational tasks, Daniel did exhibit irregularity of speech, characterized by frequent stops and starts in his speech as he was formulating ideas. Following is an example of fluctuating rate:

**Mom**: Do you want to tell Dr. Scott what happened with the DS game?

**Daniel**: (typical rate) Well, I lost it.

**Mom**: And then we…

**Examiner**: What happened?

**Daniel**: (increasing rate) Th-then (weak n) we go a DSI the- we lo-os DSI then we found the DS.

**Examiner**: So you got a DSI, you lost the DSI, then you found your DS.

**Daniel**: (typical rate) Yes.

**Examiner**: How did you lose your DSI?

**Daniel**: (slowly) I don't know.

Daniel's fluctuation between rates of speech is common in cluttering. Additionally, as the formulation demands increased (i.e., he was asked to answer open vs. closed-ended questions), Daniel's rate of speech increased, as did his disfluency, while his clarity of speech decreased due to deletions and/or weak productions of sounds, particularly at the ends of words.

*Criterion 1 is met for irregular rate of speech.*

## Criterion #2: At Least One of the Following Three Symptoms (A, B, or C)

### Criterion 2A: An Excessive Number of Disfluencies, the Majority of Which Are not Typical of People Who Stutter

Disfluencies can be divided into two categories. Stuttering-like disfluencies are those disfluencies characteristic of individuals who stutter and include part-word repetitions (e.g., "l-l-last"), prolongations (e.g., "whaaaat"), blocks (i.e., minimal or no sound comes out and the individual has difficulty moving forward to say the rest of the word), and single-syllable whole word repetitions (e.g., "I,I,I") that are produced with tension. Non–stuttering-like disfluencies are those disfluencies characteristic of all speakers and include single-syllable whole word repetitions produced without tension, multisyllable whole word repetitions (e.g., "pizza-pizza"), phrase repetitions (e.g., "I want, I want to tell you something"), revisions (e.g., "I had pizza, no pasta, for lunch today"), and interjections/filler words (e.g., "um," "uh," "well," "like"). Atypical disfluencies consist of repetitions at the ends of words known as WFDs (example: sound-ound; light-t); and phoneme insertions (inserting a sound into a word that is often not otherwise part of the word (example: be-he-cause). People who stutter also produce NSLDs in their speech. People who do not stutter may at times produce SLDs, such as part-word repetitions (e.g., "w-we"). However, although people who do not stutter may produce SLDs, these types of disfluencies tend to occur much less frequently in their speech (i.e., 1% of the time or less) than they do in individuals who are diagnosed with the speech disorder of stuttering.

Daniel produced one disfluency during rote speech tasks, including counting and naming the days of the week and months of the year. The disfluency was one part-word repetition at the start of a word (e.g., "S-sunday"). He had difficulty with accurately retrieving and sequencing the months of the year.

During conversation with the examiner and his parents, a 482-syllable sample of Daniel's speech was taken. Of these syllables, Daniel exhibited 16 SLDs, which consisted of part-word repetitions at beginnings (e.g., "y-y-yeah") of words and single-syllable whole word repetitions with tension. His total percentage of SLDs was 3%. Daniel also produced 28, or 6%, NSLDs, consisting of interjections, phrase repetitions, single-syllable whole word repetitions without tension, and revisions.

Based on the Stuttering Severity Instrument (Riley, 2009), Daniel's score places him in the mild range of stuttering (total overall score = 12). It is common for stuttering to co-occur with cluttering, particularly milder forms of stuttering. Mrs. Smith reported that beginning in kindergarten, Daniel exhibited more severe forms of stuttering, including blocks up to 4 seconds in length. She indicated that currently, Daniel's patterns of stuttering are still present but are less severe and are characterized only by occasional prolongations and blocks, but mostly repetitions. Mrs. Smith further reported that she feels Daniel currently exhibits a larger percentage of NSLDs than SLDs. This shifting pattern (from a more severe form of stuttering to a milder one with increased cluttering symptoms) has been commonly reported in children in early school-aged years.

*Criterion 2A is met for an excessive number of disfluencies, the majority of which are not typical of people who stutter.*

## Criterion 2B: The Frequent Placement of Pauses and Use of Prosodic Patterns That Do not Conform to Syntactic and Semantic Constraints

During today's evaluation session, Daniel did exhibit frequent revisions of utterances, but not frequent pauses in atypical places.

*Criterion 2B is not met for the frequent placement of pauses and use of prosodic patterns that do not conform to syntactic and semantic constraints.*

## Criterion 2C: Inappropriate (Usually Excessive) Degrees of Coarticulation Among Sounds, Especially in Multisyllabic Words

Coarticulation is the process by which sounds blend together to form words. How one sound is produced is directly affected by the sounds around it. When coarticulation is excessive, syllables of words are either dropped altogether (e.g., "May once" for "Maybe once") or blended together to the degree that certain sounds are produced with less clarity (e.g., "itslithi" for "it's like this"). It is important to note that these patterns typically occur in connected speech rather than at the single-word level. Daniel's contrast in error patterns between structured tasks on the Goldman-Fristoe Test of Articulation, Third Edition (GFTA-3; Goldman & Fristoe, 2015) and in connected speech, illustrates this pattern.

Average Standard Score: 100

Average Percentile Rank: 50

| GFTA-3 | | | |
| --- | --- | --- | --- |
| | Raw Score | Standard Score | Percentile Rank |
| Total Test | 5 | 94 | 13 |

In the Sounds-in-Words subtest of the GFTA-3, Daniel scored within the low-average range for production of sounds. As described in other testing reports, Daniel exhibited the following sound substitutions: d for voiced th (i.e., "feder" for "feather"; "dis" for "this") and f for voiceless th (i.e., "baf" for "bath"; "baftub" for "bathtub"; "fum" for "thumb").

During the Sounds-in-Sentences subtest of the GFTA-3, Daniel was asked to retell short stories told to him by the examiner. He at first spoke in short phrases. In this context, he exhibited only the same errors as at the single-word level. When Daniel was cued to tell the story back like the examiner did, with sentences, his speech intelligibility broke down significantly. Intelligibility was negatively affected by deletion of syllables or sounds in words (excessive coarticulation) and by patterns of disfluencies. The following is a transcript of his story:

"Jack and Rachel were go-go (pause)-i fishin. Ra-achel s-uh-uh-o, suh-uh-o o in a rush that she dropped her glasses and got-ot her zi-ipper stu-ucked in de jacket. Um James and Rachel hear a loud noise, it's de dog chasing the frog. Ja and Rachel caught firteen fi."

When asked to perform rote tasks such as counting slowly, Daniel's speech was fully intelligible. When he spoke more quickly, his intelligibility broke down significantly. This breakdown at higher rates of speech is common in cluttering. For Daniel, one factor contributing to this breakdown may be difficulties with motor planning for speech tasks. When asked to produce a multisyllabic word at rapid rates, many syllables in Daniel's words were reduced or deleted.

Although Daniel's specific sound errors identified at the word level should not be present at age 8, at this single-word level, Daniel demonstrates the ability to produce nearly all speech sounds accurately. Therefore, difficulties with intelligibility at the connected speech level are not due entirely to an articulation disorder, but due to the breakdowns often seen in cluttered speech.

It is important to note that Daniel's breakdowns in communication do have a negative impact upon his ability to participate in a conversation and can lead to miscommunications. For example, he mentioned something to the examiner, which the examiner misunderstood. When the examiner attempted to have Daniel clarify, he responded, "Forget it." In general, when Daniel was asked to clarify, he wasn't clear on what to do to repair the breakdown. For example, he attempted to speak louder or in a different type of voice and say, "Now, do you hear me?" Daniel's difficulties in repairing communication breakdowns and/ or in using appropriate response patterns (i.e., asking for help) when tasks become difficult are not surprising, given his difficulties with social problem solving and executive functioning documented in previous evaluation reports.

*Criterion 2C is met for inappropriate (usually excessive) degrees of coarticulation among sounds, especially in multisyllabic words.*

Overall, necessary criteria are met for a diagnosis of cluttered speech (i.e., irregular rate plus two out of three of resulting symptoms).

## Related Diagnoses and/or Symptoms Documented by Other Professionals and/or Observed During Today's Evaluation

- Attention deficit hyperactivity disorder
- Stuttering
- Word retrieval deficits/language organizational issues
- Decreased awareness of issues
- Articulation disorder
- Sample transcripts for fluency analysis

# SAMPLE TRANSCRIPTS FOR FLUENCY ANALYSIS

## APPENDIX B: READING

When the fisherman awoke in the morning, his wife began yelling at him. All you do all-ll day is fish, she said, and we never get to go anywhere. The poor fisherman-n left the house and went to his boat. He went far out to sea. He sat in the boat thinking about how unhappy his wife was. Soon he felt a heavy tug on his fishing line; he had caught a huge fish. After-r *he-he* got the fish into the boat, he sat thinking again. Suddenly, he heard a strange voice. "Please put me back into the water," said the fish. The fisherman said, "**What is- what is** that-at, I must have caught a magic fish." The fisherman thought *all- about all* of the wishes *he-he* would get.

| | *REV* | INT | **PHR** | *MSWWR* | SSWWRNT | BL/TP | PWR | *SSWWRT* | WFD |
|---|---|---|---|---|---|---|---|---|---|
| NSLDs | 1 | 0 | 1 | 0 | 0 | | | | |
| SLDs | | | | | | 0 | 0 | 2 | |
| Atypical | | | | | | | | | 4 |

REV = revision; INT = interjection; PHR = phrase revision; MSWWR = multisyllabic whole word repetition; SSWWRNT = single-syllable whole word repetition no tension; BL/TP = block/tense pause; PWR = part-word repetition; SSWWRT = single-syllable whole word repetition with tension; WFD = word-final disfluency

**Total meaningful words = 126**
**% words NSLDs = 2/126 = 1.6%**
**% words SLDs = 2/126 = 1.6%**
**% words WFDs = 3.2%**

# APPENDIX C: VIDEO RETELL

Excerpt from video retell (monologue; can also use talking about a topic of interest):

**P:** Well/and also they mentioned the Great Dust Bowl/oh *apparently/apparently* when I <u>fou-found</u> out er er[1]/apparently when I found ou(Bl <1 sec)-t about the Great Dust Bowl is that alleg- apparently since-since um/p- since people took away much of the grass that used to keep that was keeping um/ most of the soil held together/and so by the time the Great Dust Bowl ari- arose there were no more grass to be grown/so it <u>s-stopped</u> raining/and but when the wind came it was/and blew all the way to New York so/I was like s-/I was wa- especially watching my dad and I was like so basically the Dust Bowl was our own fault.

| | *REV* | INT | **PHR** | *MSWWR* | SSWWRNT | BL/TP | PWR | *SSWWRT* | WFD |
|---|---|---|---|---|---|---|---|---|---|
| NSLDs | 7 | 8 | 0 | 1 | 1 | | | | |
| SLDs | | | | | | 1 | 2 | 0 | |
| Atypical | | | | | | | | | 0 |

REV = revision; INT = interjection; PHR = phrase revision; MSWWR = multisyllabic whole word repetition; SSWWRNT = single-syllable whole word repetition no tension; BL/TP = block/tense pause; PWR = part-word repetition;SSWWRT = single-syllable whole word repetition with tension; WFD = word-final disfluency

**Total meaningful words = 92**
**% words NSLDs = 16/102 (all NSLDs must be counted in numerator and denominator) = 15.7%**
**% words SLDs = 3/92 = (all NSLDs removed from numerator and denominator) = 3.3%**
**% words WFDs = 0%**

---

1     Only counted as one moment of disfluency

# APPENDIX D: CONVERSATION

Excerpt for conversation from cluttering evaluation:

**KSS:** So then do they have any kids who need like special support in your classes/or not really?

**J:** Um/ yes/ there there still is um ACCOMMODATIONS/ um so we do have a few students/ *they don't have— they're not bound* by the same laws THAT PUBLIC SCHOOLS ARE BOUND WITH uh

**KSS:** Right/ right

**J:** IDA and everything like that/ um but we *do have a few students— I have one student* actually that NEEDS EXTRA TIME ON TESTS/ and that sort of thing/ so **they do they do** accommodate up to a certain degree/ but it's it's not um as strict as// IDEA is where where whatever it is/ you need to find a way TO ACCOMMODATE IT/ it's not quite that// strict/ *it's not—it's a little bit more/ i-the school has a little bit* more say in that/ but it's more more LIKE A COLLEGE SETUP, I'd say

**KSS:** Yeah/ the more like extra time on tests or

**J:** e-exactly 1

**KSS:** Or a quiet environment to take a test or something like that

**J:** Yes/ yep/ exactly/ and they do have an in- individualized instruction// program for um/ students *who need-/ who have special needs* and everything like that/

**KSS:** Oh they do

**J:** So they do have that **at the at the at the** school as well

| | *REV* | INT | **PHR** | *MSWWR* | SSWWRNT | BL/TP | PWR | *SSWWRT* | WFD | OC | AP// |
|---|---|---|---|---|---|---|---|---|---|---|---|
| NSLDs | 5 | 7 | 2 | 0 | 4 | | | | | | |
| SLDs | | | | | | 0 | 2 | 0 | | | |
| Atypical | | | | | | | | | 0 | | |
| Cluttering | | | | | | | | | | 5 | 3 |

REV = revision; INT = interjection; PHR = phrase revision; MSWWR = multisyllabic whole word repetition; SSWWRNT = single-syllable whole word repetition no tension; BL/TP = block/tense pause; PWR = part-word repetition; SSWWRT = single-syllable whole word repetition with tension; WFD = word-final disfluency; OC = Over-coarticulate; AP// = Atypical pause; / = typical pause

**Total meaningful words = 140**
**% words NSLDs = 18/153 (all NSLDs must be counted in numerator and denominator) = 11.8%**
**% words SLDs = 2/140 = (all NSLDs removed from numerator and denominator) = 1.4%**
**% words WFDs = 0/140 = 0%**
**% words containing moments of cluttering = 8/140 = 5.7%**

# CHAPTER 3

# PRINCIPLES FOR WORKING WITH CONCOMITANT DISORDERS

When a clinician is presented with a case of pure stuttering, cluttering, or atypical disfluency without a concomitant disorder, planning treatment can be complicated. When that same client presents with a coexisting disorder, complicated can change to overwhelming. As stated in the first chapter, cluttering and atypical disfluency are frequently found in clients with coexisting diagnoses. Perhaps less frequently, but still common, is for stuttering alone to occur in a client with another communication disorder and/or diagnosis. Finally, to make matters even more complicated, these three fluency disorders can co-occur, so the same client may present with two or three different fluency disorders that interact. In many cases, the clinician may be dealing with a client with multiple fluency disorders and multiple concomitant diagnoses.

The intent of this chapter is not to provide the clinician with specific techniques for treating coexisting disorders such as language disorders. Practicing clinicians are coming to this book with that knowledge, whereas students are gaining that knowledge about treating other speech and language disorders from other coursework and clinical experiences. The intent of this chapter instead is to assist the clinician with understanding how fluency disorders can be best managed in the context of additional diagnoses. There are myths among clinicians regarding treatment of stuttering in clients who also have coexisting disorders. Clinicians have questions about whether cluttering can be effectively treated in someone who has trouble with self-regulation due to a coexisting diagnosis such as autism. With gradually increasing awareness about the existence of atypical disfluencies, clinicians are beginning to question whether fluency treatment should be prioritized for these clients. These topics will be addressed in this chapter, and principles to guide the clinician's thinking about treatment will be presented. It should be noted that the principles are just that—principles. It is expected that the reader will follow the guidelines to adjust each client's plan for the most effective individualized treatment.

Scaler Scott, K.
*Fluency Plus: Managing Fluency Disorders in
Individuals With Multiple Diagnoses (pp 35–45).*
© 2018 Taylor & Francis Group.

| TABLE 3-1 | |
|---|---|
| **Diagnoses Speech-Language Clinicians May Treat and Concomitant Fluency Disorders Noted in Research Literature** | |
| *DIAGNOSIS* | *FLUENCY DISORDER(S) NOTED IN THE LITERATURE* |
| Autism spectrum disorders | Cluttering, atypical disfluency, stuttering (with and without affective and cognitive components; see Scaler Scott et al., 2014 for review; Sisskin & Wasilus, 2014) |
| Language-based learning disabilities | Cluttering (see Van Zaalen, Wijnen, & DeJonckere, 2011b, for review), stuttering (Blood, Ridenour, Qualls, & Hammer, 2003) |
| Down syndrome | Cluttering (Van Borsel, 2011; Van Borsel & Tetnowski, 2007; Van Borsel & Vandermeulen, 2008), stuttering (Kent & Vorperian, 2013; Van Borsel & Tetnowski, 2007) |
| Tourette syndrome | Excessive NSLDs; word-medial and word-final nonfluencies also noted (Van Borsel & Tetnowski, 2007) |
| Language disorders | Stuttering (see Nippold, 1990, for review) |
| Attention deficit hyperactivity disorder | Stuttering (Blood et al., 2003), cluttering (Blood, Blood, & Tellis, 1999; Scaler Scott, Grossman, Abendroth, Tetnowski, & Damico, 2007), atypical disfluency (Scott et al., 2007) |
| Genetic syndromes (Down syndrome, Turner syndrome, neurofibromatosis type I, Prader-Willi syndrome, fragile X syndrome) | Stuttering occurrence may be higher for those cases with intellectual disability (Van Borsel & Tetnowski, 2007) |
| Prader-Willi syndrome | Word-final disfluencies; stuttering without secondary behaviors (Van Borsel & Tetnowski, 2007) |
| Neurofibromatosis type I | Word-final disfluencies (Cosyns, Mortier, Corthals, Janssens, & Van Borsel, 2010; Cosyns et. al, 2010b) |

# PRINCIPLE ONE: EVALUATE THE WHOLE CLIENT

Following the guidelines in Chapter 2 of this book will allow you to start with a fairly good idea of what fluency disorder(s) your client is presenting with and a sound plan for hypothesis testing during your treatment. Providing specific evaluation techniques for disorders coexisting with fluency disorders is beyond the scope of this book; however, the reader is referred to Table 3-1, which provides a listing of common diagnoses where other fluency disorders may be seen. This table will help guide the clinician to areas to further explore in evaluation. Regardless of diagnosis, clients will vary in their individual presentation; therefore, all areas of communication should be considered with each client and evaluated formally and/or informally, depending on what the clinician feels is appropriate. That being said, the clinician is referred to the previous chapter to carefully consider each fluency symptom and the possible reasons each symptom may be present in his or her client. For example, it was discussed that excessive filler words could be 1) a symptom of cluttering only; 2) a symptom of covert stuttering; or 3) a symptom of difficulties with word finding. The reader was advised of some methods for teasing out the first two of these possibilities. That is, one way to tease out cluttering is to attempt to have the client slow their speech rate and see if these excessive fillers decrease or dissipate. One way to tease out covert stuttering is to observe their speech for signs of avoidance, to talk with significant others about possible avoidance, and to talk with the client about avoidance behaviors. However, even after teasing out the first two possibilities in this manner, the clinician may find that there is still a question about whether or not a language disorder is involved. It is highly possible that the client presents with one, two, or all three of the possible scenarios presented. That is, the client could be someone who avoids stuttering by using filler words, has a tendency to clutter, and has difficulty with word finding. In order to evaluate the whole client, after teasing out the first and second possibilities, the clinician may use standardized measurements of language to tease out the contribution of a language disorder to the manifestation of the fluency symptoms.

Another symptom that can be assessed informally is voice. Any gross differences in vocal quality and/or resonance will be seen upon collecting speech samples. It is important to look for differences in these areas and to consider their potential interaction with fluency disorders. For example, someone with a stuttering disorder who pushes hard against a moment of stuttering on a frequent basis may be causing laryngeal strain, resulting in changes to vocal quality. Someone with a resonance disorder may appear to have less-than-intelligible speech due to cluttering, but the root cause of the decreased intelligibility may in fact be related to structural differences that require medical intervention. Be sure to determine whether medical intervention is necessary and to gain medical clearance for treatment. Addressing medical issues also allows the clinician to understand all factors affecting fluency of speech and to therefore treat in a holistic manner. Treating in a holistic manner is extremely important, as fluency symptoms may interact with other disorders and with each other, which will be further discussed in this chapter.

It is possible for a client to present with both an articulation disorder and cluttering. When this is the case, the clinician must evaluate all aspects of speech production to determine what impact each disorder has upon each other. For example, if a client is prone to speak at a rate that is too fast for their speech production system, not only will this result in cluttering symptoms, but it can also result in difficulty with accurate production of the sounds they are having trouble articulating. The clinician must take great care, however, to distinguish the exact misarticulated sounds. A distorted /r/ can make a client severely unintelligible, and this lack of intelligibility should not be confused with decreased intelligibility due to cluttering. Although it is much less common than in stuttering, those with articulation disorders may also avoid sounds due to negative feelings about speaking. For example, I worked with a school-aged girl who had an interdental lisp and was teased about this by her peers. She tended to drop the final /s/ in words, but not consistently. My first inclination was to consider cluttering, as deleting the final sound may be observed during over-coarticulation in cluttering. But given that the client also presented with an articulation disorder, I needed to consider this complex issue carefully. To find the true source of the client's decreased intelligibility, I had to rule out an inconsistent phonological disorder (final consonant deletion), an articulation disorder, and/or cluttering. When the whole picture of the child's experience with communication was gained, it was found that her dropping of the /s/ was due neither to a phonological disorder nor to cluttering, but due to a reaction to the articulation disorder. This was a hypothesis that I developed during the initial evaluation session when the client expressed significant concern about how others reacted to her lisp. Over time, the hypothesis was further explored and confirmed in the course of therapy. I find that it is just this out-of-the-box–type thinking that we need to determine the true roots of difficulties in our clients with multiple diagnoses.

## Evaluate the Whole Client: Adult Case Illustration

Ian was an adult who came for an evaluation of his stuttering. Upon gathering speech samples, the clinician found that Ian presented with stuttering blocks of up to 5 seconds in length accompanied by facial tension and rapid bursts of speech. Upon seeing his overt symptoms, the clinician surmised that Ian's rapid burst of speech after a release of a block was just a release of tension resulting in a rapid rate. However, when asking the client about avoidances and/or methods he uses to get through a moment of stuttering, the client indicated that he tends to speed up right after a long stuttering block in order to "keep talking as long as I can to avoid any more blocks." The client noted that at times others ask him to slow down or repeat himself, which he always attributed to stuttering. Informally during the evaluation, the clinician listened for other symptoms that might be causing decreased intelligibility, including articulation disorders and/or resonance disorders. Both were ruled out. As the clinician heard moments of over-coarticulation during the evaluation, cluttering was described to Ian. He was asked if he had heard of this communication disorder and indicated that he had not. When the clinician explained the symptoms of cluttering, the client confirmed that he has experienced these symptoms. The client noted that he always felt he was a person who stutters who happens to be a fast talker. The clinician concluded that in order to avoid stuttering, the client was engaging in fast speech. Because he had a tendency toward cluttering, the client's rapid rate was triggering cluttering and decreased speech intelligibility. Therefore, Ian was presenting with primary stuttering, avoidance behaviors secondary to stuttering, and cluttering.

## Evaluate the Whole Client: School-Aged Child Case Illustration

Emily was an 8-year-old girl who came for a fluency evaluation at the request of her mother. Emily had been home-schooled since kindergarten due to teasing and an undisclosed traumatic event surrounding her stuttering. Emily presented as a shy girl who was compliant and responded to all questions, but did not expand upon her responses or initiate questions on her own. Three instances of part-word repetitions were observed throughout the entire 2-hour evaluation session. Emily's mother reported that Emily's father also stutters and that at home, most of Emily's stuttering consists of part-word repetitions at a frequency greater than observed during the evaluation session. A home video was requested. Emily's mother was most concerned about the fact that she felt Emily had been talking less at home and outside of the home. She surmised that her daughter was beginning to hide her stuttering through other behaviors, including speaking with an accent different than her own, and overall talking less. When part-word repetitions, prolongations, and blocks were modeled for Emily during the evaluation session, Emily indicated that when she was younger she exhibited part-word repetitions, but that she no longer stutters. Emily denied word avoidance, but indicated that she often has trouble "thinking of the word" she wants to say. Throughout the evaluation, Emily exhibited long pauses before saying a given word. She did not talk around the word but often sat silently with a "blank" look on her face for up to 20 seconds before saying a word. Because there was no tension or struggle, the clinician felt that Emily's difficulty was related to word finding. She scored in the low-average range on a standardized test of word finding. Her mother indicated that she does occasionally have a difficult time organizing her ideas in writing. At the end of the evaluation session, it was concluded that Emily was a person who stutters occasionally, but has more difficulty with word finding and language formulation. Word finding and language organization were prioritized for treatment.

During subsequent therapy sessions, Emily was presented with word retrieval activities, all of which she completed with 100% accuracy. Over time, it appeared that word finding was not an issue. However, avoidance was an issue. Each time Emily changed her voice to induce fluency, the clinician talked with her about using her "Emily" voice. The client would stop using her current altered voice, but would adopt an alternative behavior, such as whispering or singing rather than talking. It became evident that Emily was unable to stop her talking "tricks" completely because fear of stuttering (root cause of the tricks) was not being addressed. The clinician shifted gears toward working on the affective and cognitive components of stuttering, helping Emily to develop healthy communication attitudes. Emily did become more comfortable and spoke more in subsequent sessions. However, over time she avoided even discussing the topic of stuttering. She seemed to grow extremely anxious when the topic was brought up. The clinician felt that Emily's anxiety was getting in the way of working on stuttering avoidance and referred her to a counselor to further provide recommendations for working with the anxiety. Upon making that recommendation, Emily's mother indicated that she would not be surprised if Emily presented with an additional anxiety component, as mom herself had experienced anxiety from posttraumatic stress. After consulting with the counselor, it was determined that Emily had a concomitant diagnosis of selective mutism. Emily was considered to be most anxious about communication in general. Her counselor indicated that Emily likely did not acknowledge stuttering because in her mind, communication in general was her difficulty. It was surmised that her anxiety may have been related at least in part to her traumatic experience from kindergarten. The counselor was unable to disclose this experience, but explained that she was working on this with Emily. Together, the clinician and counselor determined that the best course of action would be to work with Emily on expressing herself, regardless of stuttering, and without focus upon the topic of stuttering. The idea was simply to get Emily comfortable talking. Had the clinician not brought in the counselor, a large piece of understanding the whole client would have been missing. Concomitant disorders are not only important to understand in and of themselves, but as these case illustrations demonstrate, they do interact with fluency disorders in a way that necessitates understanding all aspects of the client in order to plan the most effective treatment.

Note: Realize that any co-occurring fluency disorders interact and do not exist in a vacuum.

## Evaluate the Whole Client: The Bottom Line

Just as diagnoses concomitant to fluency disorders can affect how fluency disorders manifest themselves, so will multiple fluency disorders in the same client interact and present unique patterns. The clinician should be aware of potential interactions and always "study" client responses for patterns. For example, the clinician may notice that each time a client comes upon a feared word, they first try to revise their sentence, then begin to insert excess fillers, then increase their speed after they get through (or around) the feared word. Or each time the client with atypical disfluency and stuttering is having a hard time explaining a concept, the atypical disfluencies and whole word repetitions increase. Perhaps when the client with cluttering and stuttering emphasizes words more to improve speech clarity, their stuttering either improves or gets worse. Each client is unique in the way in which multiple fluency disorders interact. Only by actively studying these patterns and understanding the logical reasons behind them can the clinician help to promote the most change in treatment. For example, if the clinician notices that they see their client block frequently at pauses in sentences when learning to pause for cluttering, they should think about why this may be happening. When the clinician understands that moments of stuttering often

*Realize that any co-occurring fluency disorders interact and do not exist in a vacuum.*

occur at the start of utterances, she or he can help the client to add in fluency strategies such as preparatory set each time they need to get started again after a pause. Table 3-2 lists frequently occurring interactions between multiple fluency concerns and strategies for managing them.

# PRINCIPLE TWO: BE FLEXIBLE WITH YOUR PRIORITIES

As can be seen in the case illustrations earlier, when working with someone with a concomitant disorder, priorities for treatment and goals may change at any point from evaluation to treatment and throughout the treatment process. It may be that upon initial evaluation, a clinician working with a child with autism spectrum disorder (ASD) determines that treatment of atypical disfluency is not a priority at that time, as the client has many other things to work on that take precedence. This decision is understandable, given the multitude of issues a clinician may have to address in a client with

| TABLE 3-2 | | |
|---|---|---|
| **Examples of Potential Interactions Between Fluency Disorders** | | |
| *DISORDERS* | *POTENTIAL INTERACTION* | *MANAGEMENT STRATEGIES* |
| Stuttering and cluttering | Client is increasing speech rate to avoid stuttering and triggers cluttering. | Work on stuttering avoidance; educate client about stuttering/cluttering interaction. Once avoidance addressed, add pausing to decrease rate. |
| Stuttering and cluttering | Client is taught to pause to decrease rate for cluttering; client is having stuttering blocks when pausing. | Teach client to use preparatory set at start of each new phrase after pause; educate client about stuttering/cluttering interaction. |
| Stuttering and atypical disfluency | Client gets stuck in long stuttering block, loses train of thought, triggering increased atypical disfluency. | Teach client fluency-enhancing strategies such as pullout to get out of block sooner; teach client visualization strategies to increase working memory during distraction; work to neutralize any negative feelings/reactions to stuttering blocks; educate client about stuttering/atypical disfluency interaction. |
| Excessive non–stuttering-like disfluencies (NSLDs; noncluttering) and atypical disfluency *OR* Excessive NSLDs (part of cluttering) and atypical disfluency | Client is having a difficult time formulating, is engaging in multiple revisions, loses train of thought, triggering increased atypical disfluency. | Teach client to use tools such as visual organizers to plan discourse; teach client visualization strategies to increase working memory during distraction; educate client about cluttering/atypical disfluency interaction. |
| Atypical pausing due to cluttering and stuttering | Client is engaging in atypical pausing and is getting caught in stuttering blocks at the pauses. | Work on more natural pause boundaries in cluttering; teach client to use preparatory set at start of each new phrase after pause. |
| Atypical disfluency and excessive NSLDs (not due to cluttering) | Client is having difficulty formulating, shows increased atypical disfluency, which also increases NSLDs. | Teach client to use visual organizers for planning discourse; teach client that atypical disfluency and/or excessive NSLDs are signs that increased pausing for "think time" to organize ideas needs to be implemented. |
| Cluttering and atypical disfluency and/or stuttering | Client increases rate of speech due to cluttering, resulting in increased atypical disfluency and/or stuttering. | Teach client to increase pausing at natural phrase boundaries; educate client about interaction between cluttering and other relevant disfluency types. |

an ASD diagnosis. However, the clinician should keep in mind that ongoing monitoring of the fluency disorder is needed. As client needs change with changing life circumstances, this monitoring will help the clinician to not lose sight of the disfluency so that it can be addressed if and when necessary.

In a similar manner, a client may come to see the clinician to address cluttered speech. However, during the evaluation session it is revealed that the client is speeding up to avoid moments of stuttering, thereby triggering the cluttering. The client may have come to the clinician hoping to address speech clarity. The client may have developed a pattern of avoidance of stuttering and not be prepared to work on breaking that pattern of avoidance. Once they are educated about how stuttering and cluttering interact, the client's priorities will likely have to shift as well. If the clinician cannot help the client break the cycle of avoidance, the cluttering patterns are likely to continue to be triggered. If the client is having a hard time committing to working on avoidance, the priority may need to shift a little again until they are ready. For example, perhaps the client needs to start by reading some literature on stuttering avoidance, stuttering acceptance, and voluntary stuttering. At the same time, the clinician can introduce some cluttering strategies to reduce rate in structured activities. This might be more comfortable for the client at this stage in therapy. The clinician will need to remind the client that patterns of avoidance will lead to trouble with regulating rate. Even if the client knows in theory that regulating rate may help cluttering, they may not be able to implement what they know until affective and cognitive components of stuttering are addressed.

Whether affective, cognitive, and/or behavioral issues, fluency does not always have to be addressed at the outset of therapy. However, if fluency issues are put aside for the time being, they should be monitored and revisited when deemed appropriate.

## Be Flexible With Your Priorities: School-Aged Child Case Illustration

I once evaluated a 9-year-old with atypical disfluency who had been newly diagnosed with autism. The parents were overwhelmed with the autism diagnosis and focused on services for pragmatic intervention. Because it was thought that atypical disfluency was the least of this client's concerns to address in therapy, disfluencies were put on the back burner and work progressed on pragmatics. The client had initial difficulty joining in social interactions with others and expanding on conversational topics. Part of the lack of expansion on topics was related to difficulties with verbal expression; therefore, work in this area was deemed a priority to facilitate more progress in the area of social interaction. Several months later, the client had made progress in expanding on conversations. However, it was noted that her peers did not often listen to her, as they had difficulty following her message. She engaged in multiple repetitions at the ends of words and atypical pausing. Although focus on atypical disfluency hadn't been a priority before this time, it was felt that now the disfluency was negatively affecting social interaction and therefore warranted treatment. Her other goals could not be abandoned, however, as she still had receptive and expressive language goals to address. The clinician decided to bring atypical disfluency to the forefront of focus in therapy until the client could learn initial strategies for decreasing the disfluencies. Once strategies were learned, the clinician helped the client to use the fluency strategies in the context of addressing receptive and expressive language goals, including those for receptive and expressive pragmatics. As will be discussed later in this book, although strategies to compensate for atypical disfluency were introduced at this time, long-term strategies to assist with atypical disfluencies involved work in other areas of language.

*Whether affective, cognitive, and/or behavioral issues, fluency does not always have to be addressed at the outset of therapy. However, if fluency issues are put aside for the time being, they should be monitored and revisited when deemed appropriate.*

This example represents the constant shifting of priority that may take place when treating someone with disfluency and concomitant disorders. That is, goals must continually be adjusted to serve the functional needs of the client at the time. Additionally, if goals address the functional concerns of the client, there is much greater likelihood of buy-in from the client and the family members/significant others.

# PRINCIPLE THREE: KNOW YOUR POPULATION

The clinician is expected to treat an ever-expanding list of disorder categories. It becomes difficult to keep up with this growing list. Of course, the clinician cannot always be expected to know every population well, as this is often dependent on the clinician's exposure to continuing education regarding certain populations and/or the frequency with which the clinician may see individuals within this population in their work setting. This book will provide the clinician with guidelines for treating clients with some of the most common coexisting disorders. Additionally, the clinician is encouraged to do as much research as possible regarding the communication, behavior, and social skills of the population(s) with which they are working. Understanding the communication disorders most commonly seen in each population will help the clinician to plan an assessment and have an idea of what types of things to be looking for during the evaluation. Understanding behavioral and social profiles common to certain populations will assist the clinician with appropriately structuring assessment and treatment. In general, understanding the communication, social, and behavioral profiles associated with specific populations and pairing this knowledge with individual characteristics of each client will help the clinician to understand the whole client.

The clinician should always keep in mind the long-expressed idea that behavior often serves a communicative function (Ylvisaker et al., 2007). That is to say that a client exhibits a given behavior because the client is attempting to communicate some message. Understanding where this message comes from is of utmost importance during a treatment session. For example, a client may be communicating "I'm frustrated" or "I don't understand" by their behavior rather than by words. Keep in mind that it is not enough for the clinician to understand that their client is frustrated. Rather, it is important for the clinician to understand why the client is frustrated. Are they frustrated because they are hungry? Tired? Bored? Is the activity too difficult? Understanding the message your client is communicating will help you adjust the session's structure so that your fluency treatment and treatment in general can be more productive.

Although the clinician is warned against generalizing about any population, if the clinician is aware of behaviors that are commonly seen in a given population, this may help plan treatment. For example, knowing that a client with autism may be rigid in their thinking and need routine and structure, the clinician should be aware of providing explanations of fluency strategies that make the rationale acceptable to the client. I am constantly challenged by one of my teen clients with autism level 1 (formerly Asperger syndrome) who also stutters. This savvy client wants to know the rationale and research behind each activity; therefore, I am constantly challenged to make sure that I understand not only the rationale but also the research behind any treatment strategies I am presenting. Whereas this client requires a highly cognitive approach to therapy, another with intellectual disability or more concrete language may require that fluency strategies be modeled and presented in a concrete manner rather than explained. Additionally, those with attention deficit hyperactivity disorder have difficulties with self-regulation, which will present challenges in cluttering therapy. Understanding the potential challenges and subsequent modifications that need to be made to address these challenges will help the clinician be more efficient in treatment, which is paramount when working with multiple diagnoses.

# PRINCIPLE FOUR: ENGAGE YOUR AUDIENCE

Anyone who has had a variety of clinical experience by now is well aware that some audiences are easier to engage in the therapy process than others. For example, although a high school student with intellectual disability may need therapy strategies to be made more concrete in comparison to a student the same age with a language-based learning disability, the student with intellectual disability may be more receptive to participating in the therapeutic process. Certainly a key to buy-in is presenting your tasks at a level most appropriate for your client's learning style. That is, a client who is a concrete learner and is presented fluency strategies in a highly cognitive way will, at best, tune out and not absorb the strategies and, at worst, attempt to avoid treatment tasks. In the same manner, a client who has a high level of cognitive functioning will not appreciate being asked to imitate models of strategies without an explanation of the rationale.

In addition to understanding the specific learning style of your client, it is helpful to understand their interests. For example, if a child on the autism spectrum has a specific area of interest such as trains or ceiling fans, a good way to keep them engaged for tasks requiring fluency practice is to focus on these themes. Some professionals feel that if a topic is overused by a client, then they may not learn when to shut the topic off. I agree that a child with pragmatic difficulty needs to learn when his audience may not be so interested in their topic or the level of detail they are presenting. This is where prioritizing comes in. My clients learn that there are good and not-so-good times to bring up a particular topic of interest. We talk about the appropriate and inappropriate times to do so. Then we outline in sessions when it is appropriate to use this topic or theme to work on fluency goals. Most clinicians realize that it will be unrealistic for a child to move away from a preferred topic permanently, unless their interests change to a different area. However, if a child learns the boundaries of that topic, she or he can learn to function as an average speaker does. A person with "typical" pragmatic skills knows that they can go into extreme detail about their thoughts about the World Series with fellow baseball fans, but not with those who are less interested. Bearing in mind that the client will not move away from the topics permanently, it is important for the client to gain experience with using words on their topic of interest to 1) work through moments of stuttering with trouble words on that topic (if client is stuttering); 2) make sure to emphasize sounds in words that often become over-coarticulated (if client is cluttering); and 3) make sure to pace themselves with appropriate pausing, which can be particularly difficult when talking about topics of high interest (if the client is cluttering and/or has atypical disfluency).

Pacing of sessions will be another way you will engage your audience. For those with intellectual disability and/or delayed processing, ensuring that you allow for adequate processing time will ensure your client stays on task. When a client becomes overloaded by the content material, accurate processing will stop. The clients we are talking about require repetition, review, and reinforcement of all concepts due to multiple diagnoses. The clinician should keep in mind that it may take a client (including those with average intelligence and processing difficulties) months of repetition to understand the difference between what stuttering and cluttering are and which strategies work for which disorder. For all clients, even adults, this repetition is likely required. However, although clients with ADHD will need such repetition, unless they have delayed processing, they will stay engaged when the sessions move quickly from one task to another, as their brains are constantly seeking stimulation. Clients with sensory integration issues may also need the session structured in a particular manner, and clinicians should check with the client's occupational therapist to address these needs.

A good clinician knows that even a client who will comply with any task will find a session more meaningful if it engages their interest and learning style. In particular, students with fluency disorders may fall into the gifted range. It is important to get to know your gifted student well. Because a child's cognitive level can be higher than their social/emotional level (simply due to being advanced cognitively as compared to chronological age), the clinician must keep this in mind when grouping with other students and when planning activities. Although the child may appear to enjoy higher-level cognitive tasks, emotionally, the child may prefer tasks that are more on level with their actual age. Additionally, many children who are gifted struggle with perfectionism (Webb, 1993). Because tasks tend to come easily to them, it is difficult for them to accept when such tasks do not come so easily. When they struggle, these clients may feel not so much that they are letting you down as that they are letting themselves down. Therefore, focusing on effort level vs. performance on tasks will help the child stay engaged, regardless of their performance on the task. Also, letting the child know that mistakes are okay is helpful. Finally, staying away from comments such as, "You're so smart" may be helpful to shift the focus away from self-imposed pressure to maintain perfection. It is easy to fall into the trap of assuming that the child is bright and therefore will enjoy high-level activities. The reality is that the child will enjoy being spoken to at their cognitive level in terms of vocabulary, etc. But, surprising as it may seem, for the reasons mentioned earlier, the child may not always rise to the challenge of difficult activities as one would expect. Therefore, the clinician should be mindful of providing just the right balance of activities. I have found that starting with review of the previous session's activities, where the child knows exactly what to expect, then easing into some harder activities as the child warms up, and ending with some easier and/or more familiar activities is helpful with this population.

# PRINCIPLE FIVE: WORK WITH THE TEAM

As you will read in the next chapter, a lot of work needs to be done in the area of self-regulation when it comes to carryover of skills in fluency treatment. This is especially true for cluttering and atypical disfluencies, but is also true for stuttering. When a client has multiple disorders to think about, there are multiple strategies and overlapping terminology, which can quickly become quite overwhelming for a parent, caregiver, significant other, and most importantly, for the client. Additionally, if you are working with a client with "fluency plus" other disorders, they may be participating in multiple therapies. The more therapists can coordinate to use similar terminology, the easier it will be for the client to learn and carry over techniques. The client having multiple therapies allows for multiple contexts in which to practice fluency strategies. Parents and significant others can serve as the best reminders for carryover at home. Of course, working with all members of the team is helpful for anyone with a communication disorder. But in the case of someone with fluency disorder(s) plus other disorders, little progress will be made without the support of others. Clients will learn buzz words that apply to each therapy, but not fully understand what should be used in what real-life situation. In the case where the client may not have parents who are willing and/or able to reinforce strategies, seeking the help of teachers or other friends will be invaluable.

Working with the team doesn't mean just sending home weekly notes to caregivers. Although this is valuable, the clinician should always keep the question, "How can this person best help me?" in mind. Letting someone else know what to reinforce with a client is good, but seeking out their expertise regarding the client, the daily manifestations of any concomitant disorders the client presents with, and their knowledge of this topic area is invaluable. It is important for your client's progress that reinforcement goes both ways. If you and other members of the team have the working relationship such that you are open to discussing the client and reinforcing each other's goals on a consistent basis, it is more likely the terminology the client hears is consistent. This also allows you to streamline terminology for the greatest outcome. There may be, for example, times when terminology between disciplines may overlap and can be streamlined into one verbal cue. Maybe a child with sensory integration issues, when regulated, has decreased atypical disfluency. If so, the priority may be to focus directly on cueing for self-regulation rather than cueing regarding the atypical disfluencies. This type of a streamlined cue between disciplines will give the client the ability to make the most progress with the least amount of cognitive effort.

If the clinician is mindful to think about the whole client, how communication disorders and other diagnoses interact within the same client, and how to simplify and streamline cueing, then treating someone with "fluency plus" becomes more straightforward. Once the content, sequence, and pacing of sessions are adjusted to each client's concomitant disorder(s), the clinician is free to focus on content of whatever objectives are in place. The trick is in planning for these adjustments before sessions begin,

*...the clinician is advised to think of these suggestions as guidelines per diagnosis category. These guidelines are only useful when applied as appropriate and relevant to each individual client. Exceptions to generalizations are always present...*

expecting that adjustments are needed while a session is going on, and following through with carryover/reinforcement after each session. Flexibility in activities and approach, knowledge of what may work best for your client given their additional diagnoses, and/or integrating information gained from significant others and/or other professionals is essential.

Overall, the clinician is advised to think of these suggestions as guidelines per diagnosis category. These guidelines are only useful when applied as appropriate and relevant to each individual client. Exceptions to generalizations are always present and should be treated as exceptions.

# CHAPTER 4

# EXECUTIVE FUNCTIONING AND DISORDERS OF SPEECH FLUENCY

## WHAT ARE EXECUTIVE FUNCTIONS?

In the past, executive functions were not considered within the realm of speech-language pathology. Singer and Bashir (1999) were the first speech-language pathologists to discuss executive functions in the literature with their article, "What Are Executive Functions and Self-Regulation and What Do They Have to Do With Language-Learning Disorders?" Fitting to the topic of this book, these concepts were introduced to clinicians through discussion of language-based learning disabilities (LLDs). The specific deficits of the case study featured in this article related to difficulties in organizing oral language. Although this was not an article about fluency disorders, the client featured in the article was described as fitting the characteristics of cluttering.

Executive functions are described as those abilities that allow a person to 1) plan a task (e.g., identify what is needed for task completion; break down a long-term task into short-term projects; set goals; develop a time frame for completion); 2) organize the task (materials, support personnel, etc.); 3) execute the task; 4) stay focused on the task and avoid distractions (attention, self-regulation); 5) engage in ongoing problem solving (be aware of roadblocks and determine possible solutions); and 6) persist even when the task is difficult. There is a lot of overlap between these skills.

*In the past, executive functions were not considered within the realm of speech-language pathology.*

Populations long known to have difficulty with executive functions are those with traumatic brain injury (see Narad et al., 2017, for review) and/or attention deficit hyperactivity disorder (ADHD; see Barkley, 1997, for review). Many with cluttering have reported experiencing symptoms of ADHD. Additionally, some with cluttering have an accompanying diagnosis of ADHD. There is evidence of attentional weaknesses on central auditory processing testing among children who clutter (Blood, Blood, & Tellis, 1997, 1999, 2000). Many therapy techniques suggested for those with cluttering involve self-regulatory processes, such as regulation of speech rate (Bennett Lanuoette, 2011; Myers, 2011; Scaler Scott, Ward, & St. Louis, 2010). Finally, the latest theory of what underlies cluttering is a difficulty in self-regulation;

- 47 -

Scaler Scott, K.
*Fluency Plus: Managing Fluency Disorders in Individuals With Multiple Diagnoses (pp 47–67).*
© 2018 Taylor & Francis Group.

that is, speaking at a rate that is faster than the speaker's system can handle (Bakker, Myers, Raphael, & St. Louis, 2011; St. Louis, Myers, Bakker, & Raphael, 2007). Therefore, the link between potential difficulties with executive functions and cluttering has been long-established.

# EXECUTIVE FUNCTIONING AND STUTTERING

It is only within recent years that executive functions have been explored in stuttering. In young children, the notion of differences in self-regulation of emotion and attention during problem situations has been studied (Karrass et al., 2006; Ntourou, Conture, & Walden, 2013). In adults, the emphasis has been more upon specific skills of executive functioning, such as phonological encoding and phonological memory (see McGill, Sussman, & Byrd, 2016; Pelczarski & Yaruss, 2014, 2016, for review).

There has been a steadily growing body of research regarding temperament and stuttering in young children. Trends of these studies comparing preschool children who do and do not stutter indicate the following traits among preschoolers who stutter: difficulties with maintaining and shifting attention, increased negative emotions (including anger and frustration), increased reaction to and difficulty adapting to stimuli from the environment, and difficulties with inhibitory control (see Conture, Kelly, & Walden, 2013, for review). These temperamental features show some overlap with features of executive functioning. For example, difficulties with shifting attention from one activity to another were identified among children who stutter. Investigators

*...the link between potential difficulties with executive functions and cluttering has been long-established.*

found that those who shifted away from neutral or emotional stimuli tended to produce more fluent narratives after the stimuli were presented. It is not known whether the increased fluency is related to distraction away from emotional stimuli, distraction from over-monitoring of speech, or putting more attentional resources on speech and language formulation (Ntourou, Conture, & Walden, 2013). Although for this study, shifting attention was defined as a temperamental characteristic, the ability to shift attention is also a component of executive functioning. There are differing beliefs regarding how much one's temperament is changeable in reaction to environmental and other factors (see Conture et al., 2013, for review). Whether or not environment shapes development of temperament, it is not within the scope of practice for the speech-language clinician to work on a child's temperament. However, with the knowledge that some of these traits, such as shifting attention, may contribute to difficulties with stuttering later, perhaps the clinician can use temperamental information to prioritize which preschoolers should

*It is only within recent years that executive functions have been explored in stuttering.*

receive treatment before others, knowing that some recover spontaneously. Perhaps some children who stutter will benefit from earlier work on problem solving frustration in certain communication situations. Having knowledge about the potential relationship between fluency, temperamental features, and executive functioning skills may also help determine the best way of managing responses to stimuli within sessions to maintain productivity. For example, if a child has difficulty with transitions, sessions can at first be constructed to accommodate this difficulty. Over time, the client can learn forms of self-talk to reframe cognitive perceptions and to work through and transition away from situations that create negative emotional reactions. Such self-talk is an example of what experts propose people use to regulate their behavior (see Barkley, 2005, for review). Self-regulation involves the ability to ensure that a task is seen through to completion. Some consider self-regulation separately from executive functions, and some consider it to be part of executive functions. Whether it is considered its own category or part of executive functions, in order to stay self-regulated, you must have a degree of cognitive flexibility to engage in ongoing problem solving (see Singer & Bashir, 1999, for review).

# EXECUTIVE FUNCTIONING AND CONCOMITANT DISORDERS

The research regarding self-regulation in stuttering is just emerging. Certainly, we know that self-regulation can be a problem for individuals with autism spectrum disorder (ASD) and/or ADHD. Knowing we will be working with concomitant disorders therefore makes understanding the processes of executive function and self-regulation even more important. Likewise, although a direct link between executive functioning deficits and fluency disorders has not been established, many of

*Certainly, we know that self-regulation can be a problem for individuals with ASD and/or ADHD.*

the executive functioning deficits have been established in children with LLDs (see Watson, Gable, & Morin, 2016, for review), intellectual disability (Henry, Cornoldi, & Mahler, 2010), and ASDs (see St. John et al., 2016, for review). Therefore, because this book focuses on treating fluency disorders along with concomitant diagnoses, it is important for the clinician to understand the core deficits in executive function. Although the clinician may or may not use formal testing to measure executive functions in clients with communication disorders, the clinician working with students with fluency and concomitant diagnoses should be aware of what executive functioning skills are and what signs of difficulties in each of these skill areas look like. As the clinician learns to identify the executive functioning skills, she or he will gain a better grasp on how these skills can contribute to progress or lack thereof in treatment. For example, a client who has no difficulty with task persistence should make more progress than a client who abandons or avoids tasks when they become too difficult. Often, students who engage in such avoidance are those who have experienced significant school failure, such as those with LLDs. In a similar manner, those who stutter and who have experienced a great deal of failure and/or negative reactions to their speech may be less likely to try new speaking strategies. Finally, those who fall into the gifted

*...the clinician working with students with fluency and concomitant diagnoses should be aware of what executive functioning skills are and what signs of difficulties in each of these skill areas look like.*

category can have trouble with task persistence when the task becomes difficult. Although there may be trends toward specific types of executive functioning issues in specific populations, there will also be executive functioning issues unique to the individual. Therefore, gaining a broad overview of potential executive functioning deficits will assist the clinician in accurate identification of roadblocks to progress and proactive management strategies to combat these roadblocks.

# EXECUTIVE FUNCTIONING AS IT INTERACTS WITH FLUENCY DISORDERS

As a general illustration of how executive functioning might matter to fluency work, we will consider an example with a concomitant disorder. Working with a population of clients, such as those who have ASD, there is sometimes a "hyperfocus" on saying something just the right way. This type of focus is generally related to choice of words rather than to speech patterns. However, when working with some-one with ASD who has inflexibility and low task persistence, this can be a barrier to learning to manage moments of disfluency rather than becoming frustrated by the inability to eradicate them consistently. This type of inflexibility may also be seen in the gifted population, where students are focused on get-ting tasks right the first time (Webb, 1993). These are basic examples of how executive functioning dif-ficulties can interfere with speech fluency work. We will explore more specific examples as we address each aspect of executive functioning in this chapter.

# ATTENTION TO TASK

## What Is It?

In order to complete a speech task successfully, clients must attend to 1) task directions; 2) their own speech during the task; and 3) cueing from the clinician during the task. Therefore, initial attention to task is required, but perhaps even more important is the ability to attend to more than one task (own speech, clinician cues, organizing thoughts). For our clients then, attention to fluency tasks involves attention to multiple tasks at once.

## What Does the Research Say About Attention to Task and Fluency Disorders?

Similar to the research on self-monitoring, those with stuttering may fall anywhere on the spec-trum between not enough attention to disfluency (such as inability to identify where tension is during moments of stuttering) to too much attention to disfluency (such as focusing in on easy repetitions that do not significantly interrupt the forward flow of speech). Studies have shown difficulties among adults who stutter with tasks involving dual processing (meaning splitting attention between tasks) as compared to adults who do not stut-ter. Mixed results have been found for either an increase or decrease in disfluency when participants who stutter completed tasks involving dual processing (see Eichorn, Marton, Schwartz, Melara, & Pirutinsky, 2016, for review). Qualitatively, difficulties with attending to tasks requiring for-

*...gaining a broad overview of potential executive functioning deficits will assist the clinician in accurate identification of roadblocks to progress and proactive management strategies to combat these roadblocks.*

mulation (vs. responding to internal or external distractions) have been noted among children with atypical disfluencies. The contribution of distraction to atypical disfluencies has been questioned (Sutkowski, Scaler Scott, & Tokach, 2015). As mentioned, difficulties in focusing attention and/or shift-ing attention with changes in environmental stimuli have been found among preschool children who stutter as compared to preschool children who do not stutter (Conture et al., 2013). More studies need to be conducted to determine the specific impact of attention upon stuttering and the impact of atten-tion on fluency overall. In the case of stuttering only without a language or other processing disorder, it may be that hypervigilance leads to increased stuttering, whereas distraction away from monitoring of stuttering results in increased fluency. In the case of atypical disfluencies, where difficulties with formulation are suspected, it may be that devoting increased attentional resources to message formula-tion results in increased fluency. Increased self-monitoring has been hypothesized to be a contributing factor to decreased atypical disfluency in a treatment study (Sisskin & Wasilus, 2014). Practical applica-tion of these hypotheses will be covered as treatment is discussed throughout this book.

Although historically the definition of cluttering might imply that someone with cluttering would not attend well to a task, the current definition of cluttering considers any difficulties with attention to be a concomitant disorder. Examining some preliminary evidence that those with cluttering may have difficulties with working memory (Scaler Scott, Kidron, & Lozier, 2012), one might hypothesize that attention to task could negatively affect working memory. One must first attend to a task in order to get the information into working memory. The preliminary research with children with cluttering did not show any difficulties with attention during working memory tasks. However, it is difficult to determine with certainty that the study participants were not distracted internally during tasks. Objectively determining how common it is for clients with cluttering to struggle with attention remains a future area of investigation. For now we do know that maintaining attention to cluttering strategies in session may require frequent reminders.

## What Does the Research Say About Attention to Task Related to Concomitant Disorders?

Many of the concomitant disorders covered in this book have difficulties with attention to task. It is important to note, for example, how those with ADHD are drawn to distraction and have difficulty inhibiting responses to distractors. It is well established that the brains of those with ADHD tend to seek distraction (Hallowell & Ratey, 1994). Therefore, filtering out other distractions in order to attend to fluency strategies may at times be difficult. However, there is also research to support that those with ADHD can hyperfocus to motivating topics, activities, etc. (Hallowell & Ratey, 1994). Therefore, although it is unrealistic for the clinician to create an artificial environment that removes all potential distractions, it may be more realistic for the clinician to instead set up a therapy session that can harness hyperfocus to help the client attend to the task at hand. This involves creating sessions with the client's areas of interest in mind. Such an approach may apply to all concomitant disorders where attention is difficult.

It is often useful for the clinician to determine the root of the inattention. For example, for someone with auditory processing disorder or intellectual disability, the root of inattention may be related to the brain becoming overwhelmed by the material being presented and "shutting down." For those who are gifted, the material may not be challenging enough, resulting in the client seeking internal distraction. For those with selective mutism, the root of the distraction may be anxiety about speaking. Once the root cause is determined, adjustments in activities can be made to harness the best attention possible in each client.

## How Might Difficulties With Attention to Task Negatively Affect Teaching Fluency Strategies?

As mentioned, in order to practice fluency strategies in connected speech, clients have to attend to many tasks at once. The clinician should never take for granted how much focus this really requires. Even if a client does not inherently have difficulties with attention to task, they may have difficulties keeping in mind everything they need to do during a speech-language activity. For a child, in addition to keeping in mind the task directions, their speech, and the clinician's cues, they will need to attend to turns in a game (if one is being played) and peer comments (if working in a group).

The other piece that must be kept in mind with attention to task is the impact the affective and cognitive components of fluency disorders can have upon attention to task. Some clients I've worked with who stutter have reported that when they are in the middle of a stuttering block, they feel as if they are in a "snowstorm," where they are attending only to the moment of stuttering and nothing else. Attending solely to that moment of stuttering would seem on the one hand to be a good thing: the client has total focus to be able to apply a strategy to the moment of stuttering. However, if the client is stuck in a feeling of shame or embarrassment or fear, this may cloud their ability to access the needed strategy.

*It is often useful for the clinician to determine the root of the inattention.*

This would be another real-life case of over-focus to the moment of stuttering. Again, attention to the moment of disfluency needs to be balanced. Clinically, I have encountered this becoming "frozen" during a moment of disfluency to occur more with stuttering than with cluttering or with atypical disfluency. However, as mentioned in previous chapters, there are clients who clutter and have atypical disfluency who do experience negative feelings and reactions to their disfluencies. Therefore, this should be addressed on a case-by-case basis.

# Self-Awareness

## What Is It?

Related to communication disorders, self-awareness exists on two levels. There is a general awareness of a difficulty you may have. For example, you may be generally aware that you stutter and that this can create difficulty for you while speaking. The next level of awareness is in the moment you are facing a symptom of the communication disorder. Although you may be aware in general that you stutter, you may not always be aware of each and every moment of stuttering as it occurs.

## What Does the Research Say About Self-Awareness and Fluency Disorders?

Most individuals are aware of their stuttering both in general and during moments of stuttering from school age on. Although there are exceptions, many preschoolers who stutter are not aware of their stuttering in general. In terms of awareness during a specific moment of stuttering, I have found that most clients, regardless of age, are acutely aware of blocks or other speech hesitations lasting a few seconds or longer, but may not be aware of every moment of stuttering, especially if there is less tension during that moment of stuttering. Please remember that awareness that you are having trouble is still awareness, even if you don't have a name to put to that trouble. Thus, although a preschooler may not know what stuttering is or be aware that they stutter in general, they are likely aware that they are having trouble with speech during the moment it happens.

In terms of cluttering, those who clutter may also be aware of their communication disorder generally, but not during every moment of cluttering (Van Zaalen, Wijnen, & Dejonckere, 2011a). In some cases, clients may be aware they have trouble communicating effectively or that others ask them to repeat themselves frequently, but they are not aware that the name for this communication disorder is cluttering. I have found that my clients with cluttering are less aware during their moments of disfluency than those who stutter. This may be because moments of cluttering do not involve significant levels of tension. That being said, it is important to keep in mind that lack of awareness is not part of the diagnostic criteria for cluttering and that many who clutter may be acutely aware of the difficulties they are having as moments are occurring. This is variable by client.

*In terms of atypical disfluency, identification may not be necessary in all cases.*

In terms of atypical disfluency, the majority of cases documented in the literature describe clients who are unaware of their difficulties, either in general or during the moments the difficulties are occurring.

There is one documented case of awareness, cognitive misperceptions, and negative feelings toward the disfluency (Healey, Nelson, & Scaler Scott, 2015). It seems that when there are documented cases of awareness, the disfluency has often been pointed out to the client. Therefore, it is difficult to ascertain whether anyone with atypical disfluency would have become aware without others bringing it to their attention. Two studies discuss the idea that lack of awareness may be more common in WFDs than in other types of disfluencies. This may be due to the fact that the disfluencies have been documented with less tension and struggle than stuttering-like disfluencies (MacMillan, Kokolakis, Sheedy, & Packman, 2014; Sutkowski, Scaler Scott, Kisenwether, Thomas, & Anson, 2016).

## What Does the Research Say About Self-Awareness Related to Concomitant Disorders?

Any clinician working with clients with an autism spectrum disorder, a language-based learning disability, and/or ADHD will know that self-awareness may be challenging. Often clients can point out behaviors in others, but are unaware of the moments they engage in those same behaviors themselves. Those who are aware may be more aware that they receive feedback about their speech (e.g., "My mom always says I talk too fast") than the specifics about how they can change. If we realize that self-awareness may be a problem in concomitant diagnoses in general, it will help us understand how we may want to structure therapy sessions from day one to facilitate carryover. More about this will be discussed in the sections on therapy throughout this book. Additionally, more will be discussed regarding how to increase awareness of speech patterns in those clients with limited to no awareness.

## How Might Difficulties With Self-Awareness Negatively Affect Teaching Fluency Strategies?

Of course a client must be aware of a behavior in order to change it. Beyond being generally aware, a client must be aware of either 1) when a moment of disfluency is likely to occur so that they can apply a strategy proactively or 2) when a moment of disfluency actually occurs so that they can apply a strategy reactively. There is another consideration I must mention regarding awareness as well, especially in clients approaching the preteen and teen years. I have found that some clients are aware of their disfluencies, but have spent so much of their life being corrected by others that they have become quite defensive about them. Sometimes it is difficult to ascertain whether a client lacks awareness or is not ready to deal with the issue at hand. The issue of denial as a coping mechanism is dealt with more in the psychology and mental health literature (Ito & Matsushima, 2016). The speech-language clinician must be aware that there are times when a client is not ready to acknowledge or work on a fluency issue, but rather than stating this, will be defensive about the existence of the issue at all. In treatment, we will be talking about "going in through the back door," which is a method I use to get a client to buy in after rapport is established. By using this indirect route, the client is more likely to acknowledge the difficulty. That being said, if a client acknowledges a difficulty but states that they feel no negative impact from it, you as the clinician should explore whether this is true or defensiveness. If the disfluency does not hold the client back from class participation in everyday communication exchanges, employment at a level commensurate with their abilities, and/or social interaction, then perhaps now is not the right timing for treatment.

> *If we realize that self-awareness may be a problem in concomitant diagnoses in general, it will help us understand how we may want to structure therapy sessions from day one to facilitate carryover.*

# Self-Monitoring

## *What Is It?*

Self-monitoring is your client's ability to 1) attend to how their speech is coming across to others and 2) recognize any difficulties (such as trouble in listener understanding, trouble moving forward with producing a sound or word, etc.). In order to engage in adequate self-monitoring, your client needs to sustain focus to task and ignore distractions. A client may be able to self-monitor and identify when there are speech breakdowns in communication, but may be unable to repair these breakdowns. Therefore, self-monitoring is the step before application of strategies. Self-monitoring also can come after a strategy is applied, when a client evaluates whether the strategy solved the problem. If the problem is not solved, the client has to identify this, and has to be flexible enough to generate a new solution.

## *What Does the Research Say About Self-Monitoring and Fluency Disorders?*

As mentioned, the past literature on cluttering referred to client difficulty in self-awareness and subsequently in self-monitoring. As mentioned, current literature supports that many clients with cluttering are aware in general of their communication disorder but not necessarily in the moment it is occurring (Van Zaalen et al., 2011a). This can make self-monitoring difficult. Additionally, there is no current research or anecdotal reports to support spontaneous recovery from cluttering; therefore, self-monitoring is something that the client may have to work on throughout their lifetime of communication. Bakker et al. (2011) found that adults who clutter had a greater tendency to be "driven" to speak at a faster rate. Therefore, the rate selected by these speakers may be too fast, making self-monitoring difficult. Garnett and St. Louis (2014) found that the majority of six adults with cluttering had a more difficult time than those who do not clutter with accurately estimating how long an utterance would take them to say. The authors indicated that this finding may further support difficulties with self-monitoring among adults who clutter. The investigators indicated there was variability of performance among those who clutter even in this small sample. Therefore, each client who clutters may exhibit different levels of difficulty with self-monitoring.

In terms of stuttering, often the ability to identify moments of stuttering as they are occurring is easier for a client when there is more tension. If a client moves easily past a fleeting block or part-word repetition, it is less likely that they will be able to "catch" this moment of stuttering and apply a strategy to it. Of course, there are exceptions, and some who stutter may be more acutely aware of every disfluency than others. For example, a person who is hiding their stuttering may be very aware, almost hyperfocused upon the fact that they may stutter. Whereas some clients will need to be taught to increase their monitoring in order to apply fluency strategies, others may need to be desensitized to over-monitoring their speech. There is the danger that when a person who stutters over-monitors, they anticipate potential moments of stuttering with increased tension and struggle, thereby creating a self-fulfilling prophecy. This is not to say that thinking a person is going to stutter is the root cause of stuttering; there is no research to support this idea. However, if one is anticipating trouble and attempting to avoid it (rather than using a strategy to manage it), they may respond with more tension and struggle (rather than a strategy), which may create more disfluency. Therefore, although all fluency clients need a level of self-monitoring, a balance must be struck between over-monitoring and undermonitoring. Additionally, it is important that clients have a balance between monitoring their speech and speaking freely, and what that balance is differs for each client based upon age, task persistence, personal fluency goals, etc.

In a study of word-final disfluencies (WFDs) in 10 school-aged children (Scaler Scott et al., in preparation), participants showed decreased adjustment of their own speech in response to questions from the examiner when telling a story. It is difficult to know in this case whether the children had difficulty with 1) awareness that a question was asked; 2) awareness that an answer was required; and/or 3) ability to shift their train of thought to providing a response. The last of these three possibilities would indicate difficulty in self-monitoring, whereas the first two indicate difficulty in self-awareness. Although more research is needed, the existing findings suggest that both self-awareness and self-monitoring should be factors to consider when working with clients with atypical disfluencies.

## What Does the Research Say About Self-Monitoring Related to Concomitant Disorders?

Clients with any disorders of self-regulation, such as ASD or ADHD, have the potential to have difficulty with self-monitoring in general, and self-monitoring speech specifically. This may include monitoring for speech/communication breakdowns before application of a strategy, monitoring of the effectiveness of a given strategy after it is applied, generating a new solution when an original solution is ineffective (flexibility and problem solving), and evaluating the effectiveness of the new solution. Depending upon the severity of self-regulation deficit, I have found that some clients may need to have a "coach" who cues them indirectly to apply strategies. Cueing will start more directly (e.g., "Put in pauses") but move to more indirect prompts (e.g., "I didn't understand you, what can you do?"). Clients who require long-term assistance with activities of daily living would fall into the category of needing long-term reminders about speech strategies. The level of reminders should be faded as appropriate to help the client be as independent as possible.

## How Might Difficulties With Self-Monitoring Negatively Affect Teaching Fluency Strategies?

The reader can, of course, infer that if a client has difficulty with self-monitoring, it will result in difficulties identifying moments of disfluency to apply strategies to. Most fluency therapy does start with work on identification, whether this be stuttering or cluttering. One professional caution I'd like to make is for the clinician to consider not engaging too long in identification of stuttering or cluttering as an isolated treatment activity. Identification should be a dynamic process that changes as the client develops skills in treatment. That is, at first the client can identify moments of disfluency during very structured tasks, such as having a client identify disfluencies on a recording. At the same time clients are learning to identify moments of disfluency, they can also be working on simulating moments of disfluency to teach fluency strategies. Once a client learns strategies to manage moments of disfluency, there is little value in continuing to have them identify moments of disfluency for the sake of identification; they should instead identify them and then apply strategies to these moments. Part of the identification process may also evolve from just identifying moments of disfluency to identifying where tension is (lips, jaw, tongue, etc.) during moments of disfluency in order to adjust that tension.

*...although all fluency clients need a level of self-monitoring, a balance must be struck between over-monitoring and undermonitoring.*

There are two cautions when implementing any type of recording to identify moments of disfluency. First, some clients, especially those who stutter, are quite sensitive to recordings. Therefore, this should only be attempted when a significant amount of rapport and trust are established between the client and clinician and if the client seems comfortable with the idea. Second, the clinician should always keep in mind that even though a client can identify a disfluency on a recording, this is not the same as identifying their disfluency in real time.

In terms of atypical disfluency, identification may not be necessary in all cases. Because the research is pointing more toward deficits in language and memory that may be contributing to the disfluency, strategies may be better employed in these areas than in direct identification. This will be covered in the treatment chapters, with particular focus in the Chapters 6, 9, and 11.

Difficulties with self-monitoring might cause some clients to have trouble with identifying when an attempted solution to a problem is not working. Some clients may be able to identify that the solution is not working, but not have the cognitive flexibility to think of a new solution. These difficulties in cognitive flexibility and problem solving are integrally linked with difficulties with self-monitoring, and are common in many concomitant diagnoses, including ASD.

# WORKING MEMORY

## What Is It?

The ability to hold information in your mind long enough to manipulate that information and complete a task is regulated by your working memory. An analogy would be if you were given two numbers to add in your mind, then asked to take the answer and add another number to it. You would have to solve the first addition problem and hold that answer in working memory in order to proceed with the next calculation. When sounding out a new word for reading decoding or spelling, a student would need to hold individual sounds or syllables in their mind while they were attempting to work their way through the word. When relaying information to someone in a conversation or while telling a story, the speaker has to keep in their working memory the following: 1) What have I already told the person? and 2) Where am I going next? All of these examples illustrate the ongoing need for working memory throughout our day.

## What Does the Research Say About Working Memory and Fluency Disorders?

Some preliminary research has been done in the area of cluttering and working memory in a small sample of school-aged children (Kidron, Scaler Scott, & Lozier, 2012). No clear-cut specific deficits were found; however, gaps between scores for phonological working memory and digit recall were identified. This suggests that memory may not be evenly developed among school-aged children who clutter. Phonological encoding has been identified as a potential area of weakness among adults who stutter and clutter (see Bretherton-Furness, in preparation; Sasisekaran, 2014). Part of phonological encoding involves holding verbal information in a "phonological loop" until the specifics of the message have been planned (Baddeley, 1996). Any difficulties in this area thus far have been identified when tasks are extremely long and/or complex. Although more remains to be seen about working memory in those with fluency disorders, it stands to reason that those with deficits in working memory will require different and/or increased assistance in the development of fluent speech patterns. The clinician may or may not be working directly on use of strategies for poor working memory. Whether or not these strategies will assist with stuttering or cluttering behavior is experimental at this stage. Difficulties with working memory have also been identified in those with atypical disfluencies in an initial study of 10 school-aged children. Deficits in memory for language information were either below average or an area of relative weakness (in relation to standard scores for other testing) on standardized testing (Scaler Scott et al., in preparation). When memory scores were not lower than average, they were out of sync with above-average scores in other areas of language for the participants. More research is needed on larger samples, but the existing studies suggest a potential connection between working memory and stuttering, cluttering, and atypical disfluency.

## What Does the Research Say About Working Memory Related to Concomitant Disorders?

It is well established that many children with language-based learning differences have difficulty with working memory (see Boudreau & Costanza-Smith, 2011, for review). At least one tutorial has been written to guide speech-language clinicians in working with students with working memory deficits (Boudrea & Costanza-Smith, 2011). There are established methods that clinicians can use to assist clients with compensating for working memory deficits. These will be covered in the chapters of relevant disorders. Additionally, computer software programs targeting working memory do exist. Two of the major programs targeting working memory are the FastForWord program (Scientific Learning Corporation, 1998) and Cogmed (Klingberg, 2001). Both programs are intensive, requiring a commitment of more than 1.5 hours per day for several weeks. These programs are often conducted outside of school by private practitioners such as speech-language pathologists (in case of FastForWord) or neuropsychologists (in case of Cogmed). The research regarding the efficacy of both programs for working memory is controversial, but the clinician should be aware that this research exists, as she or he may be asked about these programs by parents or caregivers. An independent study conducted by Gillam et al. (2008) found that in comparing FastForWord to equal duration and frequency sessions focusing on academic achievement, a different computer game, and individual language intervention, there was no difference in efficacy. Researchers concluded that one possible reason equal gains were made despite the different interventions may be related to the intensity of the intervention and not the specific FastForWord program itself. When parents ask me about the potential of these programs to improve working memory and/or other processing or related communication skills, I summarize the research for them as I just have for you and guide them in making the decision that works best for their needs. Anecdotally, I worked with one client whose parent reported that his WFDs dramatically decreased after completing the Cogmed Working Memory Training program (Pearson, 2016), but did return when the family took a break from the program.

## How Might Difficulties With Working Memory Negatively Affect Teaching Fluency Strategies?

If a client cannot hold information in their mind long enough to manipulate that information, they likely will have difficulty remembering the steps to a speech strategy. Additionally, if clients with cluttering have working memory deficits, the difficulties in this area have the potential to affect two areas: 1) the client may have difficulty holding information in their mind while formulating, thereby losing their train of thought and causing them to make multiple revisions; and 2) the client may be afraid of losing information from memory and therefore be uncomfortable with slowing down and/or inserting pauses for fear they will be interrupted during the pause and lose their train of thought. We will discuss strategies for dealing with these issues in the sections on treatment throughout this book, such as how clients can learn to pause successfully while still holding information in their minds.

# RESPONSE INHIBITION

## *What Is It?*

Response inhibition can take place at two levels. The level that many may be familiar with is the ability to inhibit responses in speaking situations. For example, a client with strong pragmatic skills who notices a shirt a peer is wearing that they do not like will inhibit the response to say so. A child with strong impulse control will resist the temptation to engage in a behavior that they know will get them into trouble. Another level of response inhibition that the clinician may be less familiar with is at the level of planning an utterance. This is not something that is thought to be within the speaker's voluntary control. At the level of planning an utterance, if a message is released before it is completely formulated, the client may have to make multiple revisions. These revisions are thought to be a sign of difficulties with response inhibition (Engelhardt, Corley, Nigg, & Ferreira, 2010).

## *What Does the Research Say About Response Inhibition and Fluency Disorders?*

There is some evidence of difficulties with response inhibition for nonspeech motor tasks in adults who stutter as compared to controls (Markett et al., 2016). Links to difficulties in inhibitory control for motor tasks in children who stutter have been found, including areas of structural and/or functional brain abnormality related to cognitive control and traits measured on parent questionnaires (see Piispala, Kallio, Bloigu, & Jansson-Verkasalo, 2016, for review). However, difficulties with nonspeech tasks measuring inhibitory control did not show significant differences between children who stutter and controls (Piispala et al., 2016). Anderson and Wagovich (2010) did not find significant differences on parent assessment of inhibitory control for children who stutter as compared to controls. How these conflicting findings relate to response inhibition for speech in those who stutter remains to be investigated.

Preliminary work has been done on cluttering and response inhibition in adults. Replicating a study completed by Engelhart et al. (2010) on adults with ADHD (two different types: those diagnosed as "predominantly inattentive" [ADHD-PI] and those diagnosed as "combined type"[ADHD-C]), Scaler Scott, Bossler, and Veneziale (2015) found that the adult participants who cluttered exhibited more revisions in a sentence formulation task than controls, suggesting response inhibition. Further analysis of additional sentence planning completed by Scaler Scott, Bossler, Veneziale, Croasdale, and Irr (2016) found that those who clutter completed a sentence formulation task more quickly than controls, but qualitatively did not complete the task as accurately and had to return to the task to make revisions. Although this needs to be tested in larger samples, these findings suggest that those with cluttering may struggle with inhibiting responses long enough for accurate formulation. Anecdotally, I have worked with numerous clients with cluttering who report that messages come out before they are ready.

If we follow the logic that increased revisions might be a sign of response inhibition, then further study of response inhibition also needs to occur in clients with atypical disfluencies. It is thought that atypical disfluencies may be a sign of formulation trouble. A recent study of seven school-aged children with WFDs (Veneziale, Irr, Scaler Scott, Gurtizen, & Leiman, 2017) shows increased WFDs vs. filler words, but did not examine revisions.

It is also important to conduct a differential diagnosis when noticing that a client who stutters may engage in multiple revisions. One cannot necessarily draw the conclusion from multiple revisions that the client may have difficulties with response inhibition. This is especially true if the revisions are caused by a client's attempt to hide or avoid stuttering. If this is the case, response inhibition cannot accurately be hypothesized to be a cause for the increased revisions in this client.

## What Does the Research Say About Response Inhibition Related to Concomitant Disorders?

As noted, studies have pointed to difficulties with response inhibition in clients with ADHD-C (Engelhardt et al., 2010). In this study, adults with ADHD-PI and ADHD-C were compared to control participants on their ability to formulate sentences from pictures when a grammatical rule was incongruent with the order of picture presentation. Results showed that the ADHD-C showed more signs of response inhibition, characterized by increased revisions, as demands increased for sentence formulation tasks. The authors concluded that impulsivity may play a role in the response inhibition, particularly because response inhibition was seen more in the ADHD-C group, where impulse control is more of an issue than in ADHD-PI. If we expand that conclusion to other clients who may have concomitant ADHD or other difficulties with impulse control, such as those with ASD or learning disabilities, it is possible that difficulties in response inhibition may be a factor to consider in treatment planning for these clients.

## How Might Difficulties With Response Inhibition Negatively Affect Teaching Fluency Strategies?

If a client has difficulty inhibiting responses, as stated, this may result in multiple revisions. When multiple revisions get in the way of clients communicating effectively, whether the fluency disorder is stuttering, cluttering, atypical disfluency, excessive non–stuttering-like disfluencies, or some combination of these fluency disorders, the revisions need to be addressed. As mentioned, if the revisions are related to avoidance of stuttering, then avoidance needs to be addressed first and foremost. If the revisions seem more inherent to the fluency disorder itself (or to any concomitant disorder) rather than a reaction to the disorder, helping the client to increase pause time may assist in providing their system the time it needs to engage in planning. Allowing this time will help ensure that multiple revisions are not needed.

Beyond the level of planning, a client who has trouble with impulse control may have greater difficulty than another client with giving themselves the needed time to access a fluency strategy, whether that strategy be a stuttering modification strategy or a pausing strategy for cluttering or atypical disfluency. Clinicians will need to assist the client in realizing that giving themselves time in the first place is less work for them in the long run, as it makes their message clear to the listener. When the message is clearer in the first place, clients don't have to repeat themselves, thereby saving time. Clients will need concrete examples of how "extra effort saves me time" is helpful advice (see handout in Chapter 8). This will also apply to clients who have difficulty with waiting before following multistep directions for strategy practice or waiting to attempt to use a strategy until the clinician can present a model.

*...a client who has trouble with impulse control may have greater difficulty than another client with giving themselves the needed time to access a fluency strategy, whether that strategy be a stuttering modification strategy or a pausing strategy for cluttering or atypical disfluency.*

Often, reactions to stuttering become conditioned over time. The responses tend to occur quite quickly after a moment of stuttering. For example, I once worked with a school-aged child who had several "tricks" he engaged in in response to moments of stuttering. These tricks included first using the word "um" to restart a stuttered word, then, if this did not work, taking an audible breath and trying the word again. These reactions occurred instantly after a stuttering block. When the client was taught a new fluency strategy of pullout, he was quick to try and respond to a moment of stuttering with the pullout. However, if the pullout did not work immediately, he returned to his instant reactions of saying "um" and taking an audible breath. For most fluency strategies, until a client becomes proficient with their use, they will need a pause to access and use the strategy effectively. This will be especially true if they have negative feelings toward the stuttering to the degree that they wish to avoid or escape it. Helping clients to stay in a moment of stuttering is helpful to get them to pause long enough to access a strategy. The client I refer to had a difficult time staying with a moment of stuttering, as he just wanted to move on to the next thing (be that the next word he was going to say or his next turn in a game). I taught him to stay with the stuttering and to focus only on using his strategy. I showed him how this was quicker than getting out of the moment and having to start over again. I taught him that when it was his turn in the game, he should focus first on his speech strategy. After he had finished his speech practice for that turn, he should then focus on his game strategy and not worry about speech. In this way, school-aged clients learn there are times to be strategic about speech practice and times to let disfluencies go. Learning this type of self-regulation is more realistic for daily monitoring of speech than expecting a child to always focus on their speech during all aspects of their day. Some aspects of mindfulness (Williams & Kabat-Zinn, 2013) may be helpful in teaching this to clients who have immediate responses to a moment of disfluency.

# PHONOLOGICAL ENCODING

## What Is It?

Phonological encoding is the process by which a phonetic plan is built for a word a speaker is trying to say (Levelt, 1989, p. 12). During this process, the following aspects of the phonetic plan of the word are considered: the word's phonology (e.g., number of syllables and sounds it contains), morphology (roots, prefixes, suffixes), and stress pattern (variable based on where the word is placed in the sentence). As we formulate ideas, they move from the formulation stage to the phonological encoding stage to the stage where we articulate the message.

## What Does the Research Say About Phonological Encoding and Fluency Disorders?

The literature is mixed in supporting whether or not adults who stutter have true difficulties with phonological encoding. Some studies show deficits, others do not, and others state that tasks must be high level to demonstrate weaknesses in phonological encoding in adults who stutter vs. controls (Byrd, Vallely, Anderson, & Sussman, 2012). Similar findings have been shown in a preliminary study of adults who clutter (Bretherton-Furness, in preparation). There has been no study of this to date related to atypical disfluencies. However, the fact that the repetitions in WFDs consist of a fragment of a word suggests that studying any potential breakdowns in phonological encoding may be worthy of investigation. The difference with WFDs is that the repetition occurs after the word has already been completely spoken. However, sometimes a pause occurs before the WFD (e.g., I went to the park [pause] ark for a while yesterday), suggesting that the repetition may be part of the phonetic plan (or an attempted correction to the plan) for the rest of the client's utterance.

## What Does the Research Say About Phonological Encoding Related to Concomitant Disorders?

Those who have LLDs such as dyslexia often have trouble with phonological awareness. Investigators have suggested that what may underlie the phonological deficit is neural encoding (Power, Colling, Mead, Barnes, & Goswami, 2016). A recent study of what might underlie working memory deficits in children with ADHD found that phonological encoding was not one of these factors (Zhang, Fan, & Jiang, 2015). Given that phonological encoding is the process by which a formulated idea becomes an articulated one, it may be that phonological encoding deficits are more common in those with language disorders or language-based disorders. Verbal encoding deficits have been proposed as a reason for the difficulties speaking among children with ASD (Williams, 2016).

## How Might Difficulties With Phonological Encoding Negatively Affect Teaching Fluency Strategies?

If in fact those who stutter were determined to have difficulties with phonological encoding, it is unclear at this point how this might affect intervention. One part of encoding involves holding information in memory until an articulatory plan can be fully realized. If clients were to have difficulty with memory, it may negatively affect phonological encoding. If there were a phonological encoding deficit inherent to fluency disorders, then use of current fluency strategies may not provide complete remediation from the disorder. Whether or not recovery is predicted by inherent phonological encoding deficits may be worthy of investigation. Understanding how phonological encoding relates to breakdowns in fluency might help us better predict those who recover vs. those who persist in stuttering.

# RETRIEVAL

## What Is It?

Retrieval is often confused with memory. When someone says that their child cannot remember things, is it truly that they can't remember, or is it a matter of retrieving the information? With retrieval, the information is stored in memory but the client is having a hard time accessing the information at a given moment. If the information has been stored, then providing letter or sound cues will often help retrieve the information. Most speech-language clinicians are familiar with the concept of word retrieval and how this may play out at the level of single words or connected discourse (German, 1992).

## What Does the Research Say About Retrieval and Fluency Disorders?

Signs of difficulties with lexical retrieval have been noted among people who stutter from preschool through adult years. These signs include decreased or different responses to priming for naming tasks (Hartfield & Conture, 2006; Pellowski & Conture, 2005) and slower reaction times for tasks involving lexical access, at least in part (McGill et al., 2016). However, findings in all of these areas have been mixed (see Bloodstein & Bernstein Ratner, 2008, for review). The literature supports the possibility of "subclinical" language disorders within the stuttering population. By subclinical, investigators mean clients who score within the average range on standardized language testing and therefore do not qualify for a diagnosis of a language disorder, but who still show other signs of language challenges, such as challenges in high-level formulation tasks (see Bloodstein & Bernstein Ratner, 2008, for review). There has been research demonstrating that when compared to children who do not stutter, children who stutter score within the average range on language testing, but score lower than children who do not stutter. They also show dissociation between receptive and expressive language scores (Anderson & Conture, 2000; Anderson, Pellowski, & Conture, 2005). There is also research showing increased stuttering-like disfluencies in a group of children with a history of specific language impairment (Boscolo, Bernstein Ratner, & Rescorla, 2002). The investigators hypothesized that although the children in their sample no longer qualified (by standardized testing) as having a specific language impairment, a subclinical language impairment may exist. Therefore, subclinical language impairments may in some way be related to stuttering. Clinically, I have often found that students who struggle in oral and/or written communication but don't qualify for services may have subtle difficulties in verbal organization that are not detected on testing. Given the current state of the literature, it may be best for the clinician to be aware that a client who stutters may also have subtle differences in language formulation. Even if these subtle differences do not qualify a child who stutters to receive treatment related to language formulation, clinicians can keep the individual profiles of their clients in mind and adjust relevant tasks, such as formulation tasks, accordingly. For example, if the clinician sees that anecdotally a client has trouble with high-level formulation tasks, the client may want to practice newly learned fluency strategies first in linguistic contexts that are less demanding. Additionally, clients may need to practice in less demanding linguistic contexts for a longer period of time than those without formulation difficulties.

In terms of cluttering, although language impairments are not part of the definition of cluttering, there is some speculation that many who clutter have difficulties with verbal formulation, which is often related to retrieval (Myers, 2011; Van Zaalen & Reichel, 2015). The question is whether or not this is a true language disorder or more a disorder of executive functioning. That is, if one considers that some with cluttering may have difficulty organizing their language, then is this a problem of language or a problem of organization (executive functioning)? The field of speech-language pathology, which usually focuses on language disorders, is moving toward looking more at executive functioning skills as they relate to therapy. Similarly, the field of psychology, which usually focuses on executive functioning, is beginning to examine the possibility of language disorders in children with ADHD. The root of where retrieval difficulties lie and retrieval's role in fluency disorders is therefore currently uncertain.

For atypical disfluencies, many of these clients do have coexisting language disorders that involve difficulties with language formulation. What the relationship is between such difficulties and the manifestation of the disfluencies is currently being investigated.

## What Does the Research Say About Retrieval Related to Concomitant Disorders?

Clients with disorders of executive functioning, such as those with some type of traumatic brain injury, are known to have difficulties with retrieval (see Fratantoni, DeLaRosa, Didehbani, Hart, & Kraut, 2016, for review). Many clients with language disorders also have difficulties with retrieval of information (German, 1992). Retrieval is a common language feature in individuals with LLDs (German, 1992). When dealing with any concomitant disorder that may have deficits in the areas of language and/or executive functioning, the clinician should consider the possibility of retrieval deficits.

## How Might Difficulties With Retrieval Negatively Affect Teaching Fluency Strategies?

When learning fluency strategies, clients are often exposed to new vocabulary regarding strategy names (e.g., pullouts, preparatory set, stretched speech, emphasized speech, pausing) and when to apply strategies (e.g., proactively, reactively, etc.). This new terminology is enough for the client without a concomitant disorder to remember and retrieve when necessary. If a client has difficulty with retrieval, when the clinician asks the client to identify, for example, what strategy might apply when they are speaking too quickly, the client may know but say the wrong answer. If the clinician does not probe more deeply, she or he may think the client does not understand what strategies to use. However, if the client has true retrieval difficulties, then they do understand but are not pulling out the right term at the right time. To ensure that retrieval is not confused with comprehension, the clinician should 1) review all terminology with the client, providing definitions and concrete examples, and 2) provide the client with a written list of each term taught. When the clinician feels confident that the client has a solid understanding of each of the terms, then the client can be asked to retrieve each term (e.g., what strategy do you use if you want to prevent stuttering at the start of a sentence?). If the client is unable to provide the appropriate term but can provide it given answer choices, this likely indicates that the client knows the term but cannot retrieve it.

*...ensure that retrieval is not confused with comprehension.*

A case example may better illustrate how retrieval may negatively affect use of fluency strategies. Calvin was a seventh grader who I had been supervising in our university clinic since he began fourth grade. When Calvin came for his initial evaluation in fourth grade, he presented with both stuttering and cluttering. He also had been identified at school as having a language-based learning disability. Calvin had worked on his stuttering at school, but his cluttering had not been identified. He attended our university clinic once weekly and began to work on both stuttering and cluttering. Eventually, due to concerns expressed by his mother, Calvin also began working on literacy issues in clinic. Although Calvin had made many gains, he was unable to utilize any fluency strategies outside of structured tasks in the therapy room. One day I had Calvin's student clinician ask him about the difference between his cluttering and stuttering. Calvin was unable to explain the difference. We investigated to see if he could identify the difference given choices, but it seemed that his knowledge of both disorders and the strategies he had learned for each was not solid. He exhibited much confusion about all of the terminology. We realized we needed to take a step back and help him to better learn the terminology. Once that was completed, we needed to constantly reinforce his learning, as it is common for students with language-based learning difficulties to require frequent review and reinforcement of concepts. After this knowledge was firmly established for Calvin, he still struggled with retrieving the correct terms. This time we could see that it was a retrieval and not a comprehension problem, as he was able to identify the terms receptively. After about 1 month of review, Calvin appeared to have retained the terms. However, retrieval could still be an issue at times. Because we had now established that Calvin was no longer lacking receptive knowledge of these terms, we were able to focus on the idea that, as long as Calvin chose the appropriate strategy, it didn't matter if he used the exact technical term to name it. This is an important point to keep in mind when working with someone with either multiple fluency disorders and/or a fluency disorder with concomitant difficulties with retrieval.

# GOAL SETTING

## What Is It?

In order to set a goal, you need to 1) have a long-term outcome in mind and 2) have a motivation to set the goal. You will also need additional motivation to accomplish a goal, but the first step is having the motivation to set the goal. Therefore, the first step is for a client to have a long-term goal about why they are working on their speech. What's in it for them? What do they hope to accomplish, and why is this important to them? For some clients, this is an easy answer: there is an upcoming event involving speaking or an ongoing issue with speaking that they are ready to tackle. For others, often younger children, there may be little motivation other than that someone is telling them to do this. Finding the motivation for each client is a key piece to establish before true goal setting (other than lip service) can take place. Once a client knows what they are working toward long term, they can more easily set goals

*Understand that working to use any type of fluency strategy will be work.*

for individual therapy sessions. For example, perhaps a school-aged child with cluttering has a goal that listeners will ask her to repeat herself less (Scaler Scott & Ward, 2013). If this is her long-term goal, then her short-term goal in the individual speech session can be to focus on using clear speech during a game. For some clients, more tangible rewards will be part of long-term goal setting rather than

intrinsic rewards of improved communication. For other clients, the tangible reward is a factor in staying motivated in the short term to get to the long-term goal of improved communication. This will be further discussed in the chapters on treatment.

## What Does the Research Say About Goal Setting and Fluency Disorders?

Because motivation is a factor in stuttering treatment (see Plexico, Manning, & DiLollo, 2005, for review) it stands to reason that many clients make the most progress when they have a specific goal they are working toward, such as preparing to work toward a promotion at work or preparing to speak at a wedding. Although no research has been done in this area with cluttering and atypical disfluency, it would stand to reason that these same principles would apply to these disorders as well. As a clinician, I have found this to be the case. For example, I have worked with adults who have tried therapy previously in their lives and made little progress. When they come to therapy as an adult with a purpose in mind, they make quick progress. This seems to be because they are ready to follow through. If you think about things that are difficult for you to change, it may give you a good perspective on this. There may be things about yourself that you'd like to change, but at certain points in your life, no amount of external rewards will motivate you to put in the kind of work necessary to change this. But perhaps something changes in your life that makes you think differently about that amount of work. For example, perhaps someone has a goal to eat more fruits and vegetables but does not truly enjoy eating fruits and vegetables. Even though this person knows rationally that this is a good goal, as a young person, no amount of rewards makes them feel as if the cost of eating these foods (expense, convenience, taste) is worth the benefit. However, suppose that same person is diagnosed with a potentially life-threatening medical condition that requires significant change in diet in order to maintain health. It may be at this point that this same person decides that the benefit outweighs the cost and is motivated to put in the work needed for change.

Often, parents of children I've worked with are quick to label their child as lazy or unmotivated. I think as clinicians we have to be very careful not to mistake the client not being ready to put in the amount of work needed at this point in their life with laziness or lack of motivation. Please understand that working to use any type of fluency strategy will be work. I've also heard clinicians or parents say, "They can do it when they want to" because they see a client who is able to use a strategy sometimes in speech sessions and not at other times. Again, it is important to keep in mind that inconsistently being able to do something is not necessarily related to motivation, but to the client becoming more skilled at multitasking to complete the task consistently on their own. I encourage all clinicians to think about a time you've wanted to change a behavior or improve a skill and have gotten feedback from others that you need to try harder. Have you ever felt misunderstood? Have you ever felt that you are trying your hardest but others don't understand this? It is important to keep perspective on this. There are times when a client is just not motivated to put in the work. But when this is the case, it is often because it is not the right timing for that client. Or the client is happy with their communication the way it currently is and feels that they are having no trouble managing to talk with others. If the client is unmotivated but not managing communication well (e.g., avoiding communication), the clinician either needs to figure out a way to motivate the client or monitor the fluency until the client is more ready.

Research also shows that clients who perceive their treatment to be successful are those who believe they are in a positive alliance with their therapist (Plexico et al., 2010). If a client feels that their clinician understands their experience with disfluency and has set goals in sync with the client's needs, the client will be more likely to set realistic goals themself. If the goals are set by the clinician only, the client is less likely to buy into them. This is why it is important for the client to be involved in the goal setting process as much as is realistically possible.

## What Does the Research Say About Goal Setting Related to Concomitant Disorders?

For children who have autism spectrum disorder, goal setting may in some cases reflect difficulties with perspective taking. First we need to contrast the perspective-taking skills of two potential groups of clients with which we may work: clients with ASD and clients with LLDs. A client with a language-based learning disability may be able to understand their parents' perspective that working on their reading will benefit them long term. The client's perspective on this may differ, however. Although they can acknowledge that their parents believe that intervention will help school progress, they may be frustrated with past intervention that they feel didn't help them and therefore skeptical of this perspective for future progress through intervention. The same may be true with fluency. There are adults with stuttering and cluttering (Plexico et al., 2010; Scaler Scott & St. Louis, 2011) who have reported that they have worked with clinicians who are well meaning but do not have the training or skills to effectively help them. Although the perspective on intervention of the student with a learning disability may differ from their parents', the difference between this student and the student with ASD is that the student with LLD can see both perspectives. Due to difficulties with perspective taking, however, the student with ASD may have difficulty seeing perspectives other than their own. Such perspectives may be as follows: 1) Therapy hasn't worked before and won't work; 2) Therapy is boring and I have other things more important to do; 3) My speech is clear enough for me so why do I need to change it for others? Certainly in all cases, the client perspective is key. However, it is important to recognize some of the difficulties inherent to concomitant disorders that may have an impact upon the ability of the client to set goals.

*If the goals are set by the clinician only, the client is less likely to buy into them.*

Research also shows that children with ADHD benefit from external rewards, as they have difficulty building internal rewards (Barkley, 2005). Although I am not professionally a proponent of external rewards, I do keep this information in mind when working with a client with ADHD. In order to more effectively help these clients set goals, external rewards may have to be involved in some way. I have noticed a similar need for external rewards for gifted children I've worked with and children with no other diagnosis but who live in a household that values external rewards as part of their culture. It is important to work with families and build a program that honors their cultural values. In this way, the greatest amount of buy-in for reinforcement of skills learned at home is likely to occur.

## How Might Difficulties With Goal Setting Negatively Affect Teaching Fluency Strategies?

How many times have you inherited a client from a previous clinician and asked the child what they worked on in their previous speech sessions? How many times have they told you about the games they've played? Inherent to this is the fact that these are children, and it is encouraging when children associate speech sessions with fun events such as games. That being said, I cannot stress enough the need to have clients review long- and short-term goals at the outset of each session. Long-term goals include discussing "Why are we in speech?" in general. Short-term goals include discussing "What is our goal today?" at the start of each session. Either at intervals throughout the session (especially if a client is working on external rewards) or at the end of the session we can discuss "How am I doing on my goal right now?" or "How did I do on my goal overall?" Of course, the way goals are described should be in language the child understands (e.g., long term: I'm working on making my speech clear so I only have to say it one time; short term: I'm working on using pauses today; long term: I'm working on using tools to help with my stuttering; short term: I'm working on using pullouts today). Additionally, the discussions do not have to be labored or lengthy. For some clients, the language used for goals may need to be adjusted even more to resonate with them. Making sure a child is aware of, understands, and is on board with long- and short-term goals is key to long-term success. If goals do not resonate with the client, this will have a negative impact upon successful practice in the short and long term. If the clinician is proactive at the outset of goal setting, teaching fluency strategies should flow from here. Nonetheless, we will discuss next several other aspects of executive functioning that may interfere with successful performance even when effective goal setting has taken place.

# TASK PERSISTENCE

## What Is It?

This is the ability to stick with a task, even when difficult, until completion. This involves a great deal of self-regulation to ignore distractions, to resist impulses, and to stay organized. This also involves a great deal of problem solving and flexibility so that one can work through any anticipated (or unanticipated) difficulties.

## What Does the Research Say About Task Persistence and Fluency Disorders?

Just as with attention, we find that when it comes to task persistence, those who stutter may need to strike a balance. Those preschoolers less likely to recover from stuttering are thought to have difficulty shifting attention (Eggers, DeNil, & Van den Bergh, 2010; Heitman, Asbjørnsen, & Helland, 2004), and it is hypothesized that this may mean, in part, shifting attention away from moments of stuttering to continue with their message. Whether or not this difficulty shifting attention contributes to persistence vs. recovery requires further study.

As mentioned, anyone who has experienced failure in treatment may be reluctant to persist with difficult tasks. It is important to keep in mind that, although each client will have a different level of task persistence, previous experiences with therapy that were unhelpful should never be discounted as a factor potentially contributing to a client's willingness to persist with difficult tasks.

## What Does the Research Say About Task Persistence Related to Concomitant Disorders?

Task persistence can be difficult for any population that has difficulty with cognitive flexibility, self-regulation, and frustration tolerance. This may include such populations as those with ASDs and/ or learning disabilities. Furthermore, those within the gifted population may have difficulty with task persistence when a task seems overwhelming to them and does not come easily (Webb, 1993).

## How Might Difficulties With Task Persistence Negatively Affect Teaching Fluency Strategies?

This is one of the most important factors for the clinician to keep in mind when planning fluency therapy. Those who have difficulty with task persistence will need many modifications built into a session in order to help ensure success. Reminding clients of past successes, checking in with clients about understanding and clarifying any misunderstandings early on (before frustration can set in), and structuring sessions to build from easier tasks to more challenging tasks to winding down with easier tasks will all help with task persistence. Additionally, if a client has had negative past experiences with failed therapy, it is even more important to structure a session for success and to help maintain your client's motivation to continue to try, even when difficult. This involves the clinician maintaining an open conversation with the client at all times regarding their perception of how things are going and their understanding of what you are working on, improvements that can be made, etc.

# CONCLUSION

As you can see, many specific skills are included in the larger category of executive functioning. A lot of breakdown also can occur in these areas in concomitant disorders. Bear in mind that although we have presented all elements separately, these elements can and do interact in different ways depending on the speaking situation, your client's past experiences, their mood that day, etc. By understanding all categories and how they can break down for a client, the clinician can better understand ways to structure sessions for successful fluency treatment.

# CHAPTER 5

# ARTICULATION, PHONOLOGICAL DISORDERS, AND APRAXIA

## WHAT IS THE RELATIONSHIP BETWEEN SPEECH SOUND DISORDERS AND FLUENCY DISORDERS?

For the purposes of this book, speech sound disorders will refer to any disorders that negatively affect speech intelligibility, with the exception of cluttering. Cluttering is found under the umbrella of fluency disorders. Speech sound disorders will include disorders of articulation, such as sound substitutions, omissions, distortions, and/or additions. It will also include phonological disorders and apraxia of speech. The presence of fluency issues in clients with speech sound disorders has not been studied. However, a survey of 1,184 speech-language pathologists in public schools regarding the co-occurrence of other disorders with stuttering showed articulation and phonological disorders to be the highest coexisting disorders among the children who stutter (Blood, Ridenour, Qualls, & Hammer, 2003). Concomitant speech sound disorders have also been identified as a risk factor in persistent stuttering among preschoolers (Paden, Yairi, & Ambrose, 1999). No studies have been conducted to date examining the co-occurrence of speech sound disorders and cluttering and/or atypical disfluencies.

## MYTHS AND FACTS REGARDING FLUENCY TREATMENT IN THIS POPULATION

Because stuttering often begins in the preschool years, it is not uncommon for a clinician to be working with a child on speech sound disorders and for stuttering to emerge during treatment. When this happens, some clinicians express concern that perhaps their work on articulation or other speech sound disorders somehow "triggered" the stuttering. There is no evidence that this is the case. It is perhaps out of this co-occurrence that the concern grew among clinicians that treating stuttering along with an articulation disorder can make the stuttering worse. Again, there is no evidence to support

Scaler Scott, K.
*Fluency Plus: Managing Fluency Disorders in
Individuals With Multiple Diagnoses (pp 69-84).*
© 2018 Taylor & Francis Group.

this claim. Another possible reason for the confusion surrounding fluency treatment in children with speech sound disorders is the contrasting way sound production is sometimes treated in the two disorders. When the clinician works on articulation, they often have the client emphasize or over-emphasize sounds. Although this over-emphasis does not lead to stuttering, stuttering treatment tends to focus on gentle contact of the articulators rather than emphasized contact. These contrasting approaches can easily be blended to ensure the best treatment of both disorders. Working on accurate but gentle placements for articulation, phonology, and/or apraxia of speech should not have a negative impact upon stuttering, as long as the focus is on gentle contact. Clinically, I have worked with many preschoolers who stutter and tend to naturally use hard contacts for sound production. Some of these children had received articulation therapy in the past; some had not. Some had concomitant speech sound disorders that were not appropriate for age, whereas others only had developmental speech sound disorders. Teaching these clients gentle placements enhanced fluency. When I work with a client with a speech sound disorder and a fluency disorder, I find focusing on accurate and gentle placement of articulators strikes a nice balance to enhance both speech intelligibility and fluency.

*...some clinicians express concern that perhaps their work on articulation or other speech sound disorders somehow "triggered" the stuttering. There is no evidence that this is the case.*

It is important to note that even though there is not a known contraindication between treatment of stuttering and treatment of speech sound disorders, when considering treatment in the preschool population or in clients with intellectual disability, the clinician(s) must consider the messages being sent and make sure that they are not in opposition to each other. This is true whether the same clinician is treating both disorders or whether one clinician is treating fluency and the other the speech sound disorder(s). The terminology and cueing used must be consistent between all clinicians and between and within all sessions. For example, all clinicians and all sessions must focus on gentle but accurate placement.

There may be times when a clinician decides that it is best to separate fluency treatment from treatment of speech sound disorders. For example, if a child with delayed expressive language has been working on childhood apraxia of speech (CAS) and begins to stutter, it is possible that the stuttering is emerging because the child is growing in their level of language. That is not to say that the language burst caused the stuttering, but that increased disfluency at times emerges during language bursts. If the child is stuttering with no tension or awareness, then the best approach to treatment may be indirect treatment. Information regarding this approach is included at the end of this chapter. However, if the child is showing signs of tension in the face or body, struggle against speech, and/or communication avoidance, more direct approaches may be warranted. Information for distinguishing stuttering from normal preschool disfluency is presented in Box 5-1. At times, decreasing communicative demands upon children is recommended as part of stuttering therapy. Part of decreasing communication demands may be a temporary

*Working on accurate but gentle placements for articulation, phonology, and/or apraxia of speech should not have a negative impact upon stuttering, as long as the focus is on gentle contact.*

decrease of focus on speech sound disorder treatment. Especially if the child is struggling with speech due to stuttering, the best approach may be to focus on the stuttering, teaching the child to respond to their stuttering in an easier manner. This approach is detailed at the end of this chapter. Because it is human nature to become frustrated when something doesn't work as one would expect it to, it is natural for a child who is having trouble speaking fluently to struggle against their moments of stuttering blocks, prolongations, and/or repetitions. However, the struggle that seems intuitive often doesn't

---

**BOX 5-1**

# Preschool Disfluency—Determining When Further Evaluation and/or Consultation May Be Warranted

- Typical preschool disfluencies—indicates monitoring only
  - Interjections (um, uh, like)
  - Multisyllabic whole word repetitions (candy-candy)
  - Phrase repetitions (I want-I want a drink)
- Borderline behaviors, increased fragmentation—indicates intervention can be initiated
  - Single-syllable whole word repetitions (I-I, you-you) that sound tense
  - Part-word repetitions of two to three iterations (w-w-water)
    *Note:* An iteration is the number of times a sound or syllable is repeated, so i-i-it's has three iterations
  - Prolongations (waaant)
  - May be some struggle or tension during disfluencies
- Indicators that intervention is warranted (increased fragmentation and/or tension and struggle)
  - Increased iterations of repetitions (e.g., w-w-w-w-w-water)
  - Prolongations (waaant) with pitch and/or loudness changes (indicates underlying tension or struggle)
  - Blocks (i.e., little or no sound comes out, and child cannot move forward to the next sound)
  - Struggle, tension (e.g., facial and/or other areas of body; engaging in such behaviors as eye blinking or foot stomping when stuck), word or communication avoidance

---

help the child, but rather results in more tension, struggle, and secondary behaviors. Therefore, it is wise to intervene and teach the child an easier way to respond to their moments of stuttering. This can be done over several sessions until the child gets the idea of how to stop struggling against stuttering. Once the child seems to be getting the idea of how to approach sounds with strategies rather than with struggle, the clinician can return to work on the speech sound disorder, incorporating fluency strategies into the intervention as needed. I have found that when children are exhibiting a lot of tension and struggle, even if they are very young or they have a diagnosis of intellectual disability, they tend to respond quickly to strategies that will help them get the words out easier. I have observed that the hardest clients to achieve carryover of fluency strategies are those whose stuttering seems to hold them back the least. For example, a child who has easy part-word repetitions, is not always aware of the repetitions, and doesn't let the repetitions stop them from talking, may not want to put in the work needed to use strategies in response to stuttering. This makes logical

*There may be times when a clinician decides that it is best to separate fluency treatment from treatment of speech sound disorders.*

sense; if there is little impact from my stuttering, why am I spending time with strategies when I could be spending playing, talking, and having fun? For those children who experience longer blocks that hinder their speech, often I find that they will quickly learn strategies such as "rainbow speech" (see detail in Activity 5-3 and at end of Chapter 6 for intellectual disability) and incorporate these strategies into real moments of stuttering. Children will vary in their response to teaching direct strategies, but when the clinician sees that the client can at least respond to cues in session to use fluency strategies appropriately, it signifies that it is a good time to restart work on speech sound disorders along with fluency treatment.

# WHAT EXECUTIVE FUNCTIONING ISSUES CAN I EXPECT WITH SPEECH SOUND DISORDERS?

When the clinician is working with speech sound disorders in preschoolers, there will be differences in levels of self-regulation than in older clients. One message that is important about self-regulation is the idea that for preschoolers, moments of frustration are just simply moments rather than something the preschooler holds onto long term. Therefore, although it is important to address negative attitudes toward speaking as early as they appear, clinicians should not be too concerned if children experience moments of frustration. This is also good information to pass along to parents, who may feel their child's frustration longer than their child actually does. Because self-regulation skills are still developing in preschoolers, clinicians must keep this in mind when considering the child's ability to self-monitor and apply strategies accordingly. Additionally, if a child has a concomitant diagnosis that has at its core difficulties with self-regulation (such as autism spectrum disorder or attention deficit hyperactivity disorder), expectations for self-regulation should be adjusted accordingly.

There are no executive functioning issues that are inherent to speech sound disorders. However, some children with CAS may have additional learning challenges, which may bring with them difficulties in working memory and/or attention. See Chapters 6, 7, and 8 for strategies regarding these areas. The most difficult area for clients working on articulation and fluency may be self-regulation related to emphasis of sounds. As mentioned, when working on correct articulation of sounds, clients may be taught to and/or inadvertently emphasize these sounds when speaking. The emphasis demonstrates awareness and carryover, which is normally a clinician's dream when it comes to generalization of skills. However, as mentioned, this over-emphasis is often not fluency enhancing. Teaching the client gentle but accurate placement of the articulators is the balance the client must learn to move forward in both fluency and articulation therapy.

If your client is cluttering and has difficulty with articulation, they will not experience the conflict between hard contact of articulators for articulation and gentle contact for fluent speech. Rather, harder contact will lead to emphasis of speech sounds, which should increase speech clarity in terms of both articulation and cluttering. Likewise, including all parts of words when working on phonological processes such as weak syllable deletion will help to increase clarity for cluttering.

# CHILDHOOD APRAXIA OF SPEECH AND INCONSISTENT SPEECH SOUND DISORDER

## *Core Vocabulary*

One approach that is often recommended for children with inconsistent speech sound disorder, including inconsistent phonological disorders, is to focus on core vocabulary (Dodd, Holm, Crosbie, & McIntosh, 2006). Whereas Dodd and colleagues (2006) differentiate this approach from those used with CAS, Bernthal, Bankson, and Flipsen, Jr. (2012) propose that some children with CAS may benefit from components of a core vocabulary approach.

Core vocabulary focuses on consistency rather than accuracy of speech sound production. The goal is to increase overall consistency of speech sound production patterns so that the productions 1) are more intelligible to the child's communication partners and 2) are more stimulable for future intervention. For children with inconsistent phonological disorders, a list of 50 functional vocabulary words is generated with the help of parents and teachers. These may include multisyllabic words from the start. The child's best productions of each syllable in each word are elicited, and consistency of production is reinforced through drills (Dodd et al., 2006).

For those clients with CAS, Bernthal et al. (2012) recommend the same concept of choosing functional words for the child. However, instead of drills on individual syllables, children with CAS need to focus on transition between sounds, such as labial to alveolar (e.g., "bunny"). Bernthal et al. (2012) suggest choosing categories of words (such as animals) that lend themselves to practice at one-, two-, and three-syllable levels.

For clients who are working on stuttering, add rainbow speech to start words gently and easily. Any approach that the clinician finds is effective (e.g., core vocabulary, backwards buildup, phonological contrasts, etc.) for their clients with speech sound disorders can be combined with fluency-enhancing strategies to address both disorders concurrently.

# PHONOLOGICAL DISORDERS, THE CYCLES APPROACH, AND FLUENCY STRATEGIES

The cycles approach (Hodson & Paden, 1983) is often recommended in treatment of clients presenting with multiple phonological process errors. In this approach, several phonological error patterns are selected as initial goals. Each session (or week if multiple sessions occur in one week), one of these error patterns is focused on. For example, suppose the clinician decided that the client needed to work on the following four phonological error patterns: final consonant deletion, weak syllable deletion, stopping, and backing. The linguistic context in which each process is addressed advances as the client advances. Therefore, the client may be working at one linguistic level for one process and another linguistic level for another process. The schedule of treatment would look something like this:

- Week 1: Final consonant deletion (single-word level)
- Week 2: Weak syllable deletion (phrase level)
- Week 3: Stopping (single-word level)
- Week 4: Backing (sentence level)
- Week 5: Final consonant deletion (phrase level)
- Week 6: Weak syllable deletion (phrase level)
- Week 7: Stopping (single-word level)
- Week 8: Backing (sentence level)

As you can see from this example, the client meets the criteria after week one to move on to working on final consonant deletion at the phrase level the next time in the cycle this process is addressed (week 5). For all other phonological process errors, the client continues at the level on which they started (the next time that cycle occurs) until they are ready to move on to the next level.

Remember that fluency strategies can be used as needed. For example, when a client is working on final consonant deletion (FCD), they can use a gentle stretch on the word "beeeed" (see Activity 5-3), gently emphasizing the final sound to address the FCD as well. Or if working at the phrase level they might say "Goooo to bed." Table 5-1 illustrates ways of combining the cycles approach with fluency-enhancing strategies.

| | TABLE 5-1 | | | |
|---|---|---|---|---|
| **Combining the Cycles Approach With Fluency-Enhancing Strategies** | | | | |
| WEEK | PHONOLOGICAL PROCESS TARGETED | LINGUISTIC LEVEL | RAINBOW SPEECH | LIGHT CONTACT |
| 1 | Final consonant deletion | Single word | Beeed | Gentle touch of lips for /b/ in "bed" |
| 2 | Weak syllable deletion | Phrase | Waaant tomato | Gentle touch of tongue to teeth for /t/ in "tomato" |
| 3 | Stopping | Single word | Fuuun | Gentle touch of top teeth to bottom lip for /f/ in "fun" |
| 4 | Backing | Sentence | IIII want toooo go home | Gentle touch of back tongue to roof of mouth for /g/ in "go" |

# PHONOLOGICAL PROCESS DISORDERS, THE LINGUISTIC BASE, AND FLUENCY

If a client exhibits a pure phonological process error, they have a misunderstanding of the rule for producing the word. We know that often a child has this misunderstanding, but also has difficulty with motor production of the word. First what must be addressed in treatment is making sure that the client understands the concept behind the error they are making. Here is an example for final consonant deletion for which the concept is "words have endings":

- Do you know what a body part is? How many body parts can you name? They are parts that you put together to make your whole body. Did you know that words have parts too? We can clap out the parts. Listen. "po—ta—to" (clinician claps hands together as says each syllable). You try it. Let's see if we can figure out how many parts your name has. Let's try some others (they may have to just listen to you clap first to name the number of parts; if needed you can have them count the claps).
- Now we've figured out the big parts to words. But words have even smaller parts—they are called sounds. You might know sounds—they go with letters. What sound does "b" make? What letter does your name start with? I bet you know what sound that letter makes!
- Let's see if we can tell how many sounds these words have. (Present three to four sounds to start) I am going to clap each time I make a sound, and you tell me how many times I clap.
  - b-e-d; c-a-t; d-o-g; i-n; f-i-sh
- Now let's see if you can clap when I say the sounds (may have to clap together at first, then fade to child clapping on their own).
- Okay, you are getting good at hearing all the sounds in words. Now let's see if you can hear just the last sound in a word. I'm going to say it a little louder than the others. Listen and see if you can hear it.
  - b-e-**d**; c-a-**t**; f-i-**sh**
- Great, now you can hear the last sound. The word would sound silly if I left the last sound out. Listen, here's "fish": f-i; here's "cat": c-a
- Now see if you can tell when I leave the sound off or not. Sometimes I will and sometimes I won't. Don't let me trick you!

| TABLE 5-2 | | |
|---|---|---|
| **Phonological Process Concepts to Introduce** | | |
| *PROCESS* | *CONCEPT* | *INCORPORATE FLUENCY STRATEGIES* |
| Final consonant deletion | Words have endings | Use light contact to emphasize ending sound. |
| Stopping | "Stop" vs. "go" sounds | Gentle placement of articulators to get air moving; stretch into vowel or syllable with rainbow speech as needed (e.g., for "sock" use gentle placement of tongue on alveolar ridge, begin /s/ with gentle air and use rainbow speech or stretch on "o", "sooooock"). |
| Cluster reduction | All letters go to work and make a sound | If client becomes blocked on clusters as in "stripe," use light contact to approach sounds in the cluster. Blow out a little air while making sounds to get sounds moving. Continue stretching the vowel with rainbow speech if needed: "striiiipe." |
| Weak syllable deletion | Words must have all their parts | Use light contact to emphasize missing syllable, use rainbow speech to stretch vowel if needed (e.g., tomaaato). |
| Metathesis | Sounds must be said in the right order<br><br>Concrete cue: Put socks on before shoes or will look "funny" | Use rainbow speech on each part of word during backward chaining, as described in Activity 5-4. |
| Epenthesis | If there are too many sounds, the word will sound "funny" | Use light contact to place articulators and transition to next sound. For example, gently produce the lip posture for /b/, gently lift tongue tip up then attempt "blue." Use rainbow speech to stretch vowel if needed: "bluuue." |

As this example illustrates, making the concept of the linguistic rule the child needs to learn concrete is key to addressing the phonological process error. Table 5-2 provides a list of common phonological process errors, the concept that needs to be taught regarding that error, and suggestions for incorporating fluency strategies into work on these concepts.

The remainder of this chapter covers activities for management of fluency and speech sound disorders. Included are indirect strategies to use with preschoolers, activities to regulate hard vs. light contact, and activities to increase awareness of articulators for accurate speech sound production while using fluency strategies. Also included are activities that facilitate practice with rainbow speech and light contact. Finally, activities for work on metathesis and backward chaining, and apraxia of speech and Dynamic Temporal and Tactile Cueing for Speech Motor Learning (DTTC) are presented in combination with use of fluency strategies.

## *Additional Means for Building Transitions Between Sounds*

Touch cues are often recommended for transitions between sounds in CAS. See Bashir, Grahamjones, and Yale Bostwick (1984) for further information. All touch cues should be accurate and gentle to facilitate accuracy of production and speech fluency. If clients use these to self-cue, be sure they are not becoming a secondary behavior or "trick" to facilitate fluency. With a disfluent child prone to tricks, the clinician may want to use the touch cues on the child, but not have them self-cue.

| TABLE 5-3 | | | |
|---|---|---|---|
| **Example of Combining CAS With Fluency Approaches** | | | |
| *LEVEL OF DTTC* | *TARGET WORD: "BUNNY"* | *FLUENCY CUES* | *CAS CUES* |
| Simultaneous production | Say in unison; clinician fades cues until child says accurately alone. | Light contact of articulators, see Activities 5-1 and 5-6; simultaneous production will be fluency enhancing. | Visual cues as in Activity 5-6; add rainbow speech to enhance slowed rate as needed. |
| Immediate repetition | Auditory and visual model | Light contact and neutral as in Activity 5-7 as needed | Add touch or gestural cues as needed. |
| Repetition after delay | Delay of 1 to 2 seconds before child imitates; once successful child repeats several times in a row. | Light contact and neutral as in Activity 5-7 as needed | Go back a level until get to level of perfect practice. |
| Spontaneous production | Ultimate goal in DTTC but avoid incorrect practice | Light contact and neutral as in Activity 5-7 as needed | Go back a level until get to level of perfect practice. |

DTTC (Strand, Stoeckel, & Bass, 2006) is a system of cueing often used to facilitate movement between sounds in treating CAS. When implementing DTTC, the treating clinician moves the client through four levels of a speech production hierarchy: simultaneous production, immediate repetition, repetition after delay, and spontaneous production. The treatment method is considered dynamic in that the clinician may move back and forth with a client between levels to ensure that the client is engaging in perfect practice of targets rather than continued incorrect practice. See Maas, Gildersleeve-Neumann, Jakielski, & Stoeckel (2014) and McCauley & Strand (2008) for further description of approaches to CAS and evidence base for each approach. Please see Table 5-3 for integration of DTTC with fluency treatment.

# INFORMATION FOR PARENTS AND TEACHERS ON AN INDIRECT APPROACH TO TREATMENT

When speaking to the child or around him or her (i.e., when she or he is within earshot), use the strategies described here. These strategies have been shown to decrease the pace of the communication interaction. This tends to result in increased time for formulation that many preschoolers need. As a result, it increases fluency of speech.

The child at whom these strategies are targeted may or may not imitate the strategies directly. It is okay if they do, and okay if they do not imitate them. We don't comment to the child on his response either way. The strategies are indirect and produced by the adults around the child.

What we are most looking for is a decrease in disfluency overall, but especially a decrease in fragmented speech (such as repeating a sound or syllable, like th-th-that, or ba-baby) and/or a decrease in any tension heard during speech (such as a tense "uh-uh I am five years old"). We are also looking for a decrease in the number of repetitions of a word, sound, or syllable (e.g., a-and rather than a-a-a-a-and; ba-baby rather than ba-ba-ba-ba-baby). If we see these types of decreases, that is a sign that the strategies are working. We may also see an increase in typical preschool disfluencies that do not indicate stuttering, such as phrase repetitions (I want, I want) or interjections (um, uh). An increase in these type of disfluencies is also a sign that the strategies are working, as the child is moving from stuttering-like disfluencies (i.e., more fragmented and more tense) to typical preschool disfluencies (i.e., less fragmented, repetitions of larger chunks of information, and less tense).

Please implement the strategies and monitor the child's progress closely. This will help us intervene further if needed.

## Strategy One: Increased Use of Pausing in Your Speech

Speak with increased pauses in your speech. Your speech should not be slower or more stretched out; it should just contain an increased amount of pauses from what you may normally use. This strategy is often referred to as "Mr. Roger's Speech."

**Example**: When we go home/we can/build with blocks.

(/ indicates a pauses).

**Note**: There is no exact place you must pause; everyone's pattern will be a little different. The goal is just to increase the pausing. These speech patterns are a new habit and hard to change, so go easy on yourself. Start by using them during book reading (when it is quieter and you don't have to think about pausing and formulating), and gradually work pauses more and more into your daily speech as you are able.

## Strategy Two: Delayed Response

When your child asks a question or makes a comment to which you'd like to respond, count in your head to two (i.e., "one, two") before responding. If the child is commenting during play, you count, and the child continues talking, continue to count to two until your child has finished what they are saying. Then add your answer or comment, using the pausing in Strategy One in your comment as well.

**Note**: I sometimes find it helpful to physically count to two with my fingers behind my back to help remind me to use this strategy.

## Strategy Three: Modified Questions

Instead of asking a question, you rephrase it in an indirect manner (e.g., rather than "What is that?" you say, "**I wonder**/if you know/what that is" or "**I'll bet**/you can name/that dinosaur"; rather than "What do you want to play?", you can say, "**Maybe**/we should play/dinosaurs next" or "**I think**/you might like/to go outside").

**Note**: This does not mean you will never ask your child questions. It's just a way to give the child an opportunity to respond without the time pressure that questions can produce.

# ACTIVITY 5-1:
# LIGHT VERSUS GENTLE CONTACT

**For the speech clinician**: Model hard and light contact using the following examples. Focus on the contrast between "hard" and "gentle" or "light" touch of the articulators for the beginning sounds. Feel free to use pictures, stuffed animals, games, etc., to get the concepts across.

## *Hard Sounds and Gentle Sounds*

When we say sounds, we can say them in a hard way, like this:

- Fish

- Snake

- Whale

- Penguin

- Kangaroo

Or we can touch our teeth, lips, and tongue together gently and say the sounds like this:

- Fish

- Snake

- Whale

- Penguin

- Kangaroo

# ACTIVITY 5-2:
# MY SPEECH SOUND(S)

Here's how I say my speech sound(s):



My speech sound is  _____



I use my (please circle all that apply):

   Lips

   Tongue

   Teeth


With my lips, I _____



With my tongue, I _____



With my teeth, I _____

# ACTIVITY 5-3:
# I MAKE MY SOUNDS GENTLY WITH RAINBOW SPEECH

Rainbow Speech Practice With My Speech Sounds (please refer to Activity 6-2)

**Note:** "Rainbow speech" can be changed to other names that resonate with your client, such as "easy speech," "stretched speech," etc.

**Directions:** Choose seven colors to draw a rainbow in the space below. As you draw each arc of the rainbow, say the word that starts with the speech sound you are working on. Remember to stretch the vowel in the word until you get to the end of the rainbow (e.g., "daaaad").

List of words to practice (to be filled in by your speech teacher):

Draw your rainbow here:

# ACTIVITY 5-4:
# BACKWARD CHAINING AND FLUENCY PRACTICE—INTRODUCTION

Although some literature proposes the use of backward chaining with CAS (Velleman, 1998), there has been debate about whether breaking up a word in this manner impedes smooth movement between sounds, which is the goal of treatment for CAS. I have found backwards chaining to be especially effective for school-aged children who present with the phonological process of metathesis. When using this with a client who stutters, it is important to keep in mind that stuttering blocks may occur at the start of phonation. Therefore, when using backward chaining, the client may want to use rainbow speech for the initiation of each syllable. For example:

Elephant

In backward chaining, the child says:

- Phant

- Lephant

- Elephant


When working with a client on metathesis and stuttering, the clinician may want to add rainbow speech:

- Phaaant

- Leeephant

- Eeeelephant

# ACTIVITY 5-5:
# BACKWARD CHAINING AND FLUENCY PRACTICE

**Directions**: Determine 10 multisyllabic words that work well for your client's core vocabulary or that your client struggles with. For each word, print a picture and cut it into thirds: front third, middle third, back third. You can use the actual letters of each syllable if the child is a reader or just parts of the picture if the child is not a reader.

**Say**: Let's put the pieces together to say the words. We will go from the back to the front of each word. As we put out each piece of the word/picture, let's move our finger under it, like this (demonstrate moving finger left to right under letters of the word or just under the picture). We will use our rainbow speech when we say each part of the word.

**Example**:
- (back third of butterfly)
  Flyyyyy (moving finger from left to right under letters or picture)

- (middle third of butterfly)
  Teeerfly (moving finger from left to right under letters or picture of both parts of word)

- (front third of butterfly)
  Buuuuterfly (moving finger from left to right under letters or picture of all parts of word)

**Note**: Because clients may have difficulty with the transitions between sounds and because stuttering blocks often occur at the start of a word or syllable, using rainbow speech on only the first syllable of the multisyllabic word may not be enough. If this is the case, help the client with the transition between syllables by having them extend the vowel from the previous syllable until they can transition to producing the next syllable.

**Example**:
- Teeeeeeeerfly (don't stop holding "er" until they can start to say "fly")

- Buuuuuuuuuteeeerfly (don't stop holding "uh" until they can start to say "ter"; don't stop holding "er" until they can transition to "fly")

# ACTIVITY 5-6:
# CUES FOR ADJUSTING TENSION FOR
# FLUENCY AND PLACEMENT OF ARTICULATORS

**Note to the clinician**: These client-created descriptions of how sounds get stuck in stuttering and strategies for getting them unstuck can also be applied to cueing to transition between sounds in words for CAS. Use Activity 5-7 "Going to neutral" and gentle contact of articulators for clients who are stuck due to stuttering blocks. Add touch cues and DTTC methods for children with CAS.

## Cues for Adjusting Tension for Fluency and Placement of Articulators

| LETTERS/SOUNDS | WHERE SOUND GETS STUCK | NAME OF VILLAIN (CAUSING SOUNDS TO GET STUCK) | NAME OF HERO (UNLOCKING SOUNDS OR HELPING SOUNDS BE CLEAR) |
|---|---|---|---|
| p, b, m, w | Lips | Lip Locker | Gentle Unlocker |
| k, c (making /k/ sound), g | Back of tongue | Back Tonguer | Back Releaser |
| f, v | Lips and teeth | Tooth-Lip | Lip Releaser |
| th | Teeth and tongue | Tongue Trapper | Tongue Releaser |
| h and vowels | Throat (go to neutral then apply rainbow speech) | Throat Attacker | Neutralizer |
| t, d, s, z, n, l | Tongue tip against bottom or top teeth | Tooth-Tonguer | Tip Releaser |
| j, sh, ch, r, y | Sides of tongue | Tongue Sideliner | Side Releaser |

# ACTIVITY 5-7:
## GOING TO NEUTRAL

When stuttering happens, it is normal to want to try to fight it and push the sound out.

But when you fight stuttering, it fights back harder.

So if you go to neutral then you stop the fight, you can have control and use a strategy again.

Neutral means you put your lips so that they are just touching or barely touching and nothing is happening. You are not trying to push a sound out, and you are not doing anything with your lips.

When you are sure your lips are in neutral, then try to stretch the first vowel (rainbow speech) to get the word out.

You can use neutral when a stretch doesn't seem to be working. Or if you are stuck on a vowel or /h/ sound.

Remember if you try neutral and the sound still gets stuck, keep going back to neutral until you can get the sound out. It will take a little practice but will get easier. It will help you have control to say what you want.

Sometimes you can use only neutral and then say the word you were stuck on. If you still get stuck, add the stretch on the vowel of the difficult word.

# CHAPTER 6

# INTELLECTUAL DISABILITY

## WHAT FLUENCY DISORDERS ARE MORE COMMONLY FOUND IN THIS POPULATION?

Fluency disorders are frequently occurring in individuals with intellectual disability (ID; Van Borsel & Tetnowski, 2007). ID is a neurodevelopmental disorder whereby the client presents with both challenges in intellectual and adaptive functioning (American Psychiatric Association, 2013). The typical intelligence quotient (IQ) score on standardized tests for someone with ID is approximately 70 to 75 or lower. ID may be associated with a specific syndrome or be nonspecific. It is thought that fluency disorders may present more frequently in clients with ID and that greater degrees of ID may be related to higher levels of disfluency (see Van Borsel & Tetnowski, 2007, for review). Fluency disorders have been identified in genetic syndromes, many of which include individuals with ID. Van Borsel and Tetnowski (2007) reviewed the literature regarding documentation of disfluency in six genetic syndromes. Types of disfluency documented within these syndromes included stuttering with and without secondary behaviors, atypical disfluency, excessive non–stuttering-like disfluencies (NSLDs), and/or cluttering. The authors noted stuttering-like disfluencies (SLDs) with and without secondary behaviors, NSLDs, and cluttering in individuals with Down syndrome, a genetic disorder that may or may not result in ID. Those with fragile X syndrome (FXS), the most common genetic cause of ID and often associated with autism (Cohen et. al, 2005), are considered to have a higher occurrence of SLDs than those with general ID, but lower occurrence than those with Down syndrome. Those with FXS have been noted to present with a rapid rate of speech (Belser & Sudhalter, 2001), although cluttering has not been formally studied in this population. Van Borsel and Tenowski (2017) reported SLDs without secondary behaviors and word-final disfluencies (WFDs) in Prader Willi syndrome, a genetic syndrome that leads to ID, behavior disorders, and obesity (Dykens, Roof, & Hunt-Hawkins, 2017). The researchers also noted that in Tourette syndrome, a disorder characterized by chronic motor and vocal tics (American Psychiatric Association, 2013), there are fewer instances of SLDs and more repetition of phrases and whole words

Scaler Scott, K.
*Fluency Plus: Managing Fluency Disorders in
Individuals With Multiple Diagnoses (pp 85-107).*
© 2018 Taylor & Francis Group.

(rather than parts of words as seen in WFDs) at the ends of clauses. WFDs (both repetitions and prolongations), cluttering, and stuttering blocks have been identified in neurofibromatosis type I (Cosyns et al., 2010; Cosyns, Mortier, Corthals, Janssens, & Van Borsel, 2010). It should be noted that not all cases of these genetic syndromes will present with ID and that disfluency in genetic syndromes may share the same characteristics as disfluency in the general population (Van Borsel & Tetnowski, 2007).

# MYTHS AND FACTS REGARDING FLUENCY TREATMENT IN THIS POPULATION

One myth that needs to be addressed is the idea that if someone is not of average cognitive ability, they cannot learn fluency strategies. It is true that those with ID may need more repetition and reinforcement of concepts than those without ID. It is true that strategies may take longer to teach in the ID population than in clients without ID. However, this does not mean that the client is incapable of learning to use fluency strategies. It also does not mean that the client is incapable of using fluency strategies in real-life situations. What may need to be different in a client with ID is the clinician's (and family's) definition of success. That is, clients with ID may have a harder time with online monitoring of speech skills without cues. But they may be able to monitor speech with cues from an appropriate person. I tell my clients' families to expect that more support will likely be needed in self-monitoring. That is, the client will learn the strategy, but may apply it more frequently when others can "coach" them with a verbal or nonverbal reminder to apply it.

Another myth related to this population is the idea that even if they are stuttering with secondary behaviors, clients with ID are largely unaware of their stuttering and therefore do not experience any difficulties with the affective and cognitive components of stuttering. I have worked with numerous clients with ID who experience these components. The difference often is in how the components manifest themselves. For example, a client who does not have ID might be able to describe their stuttering as "frustrating." Some clients (though of course not all) with ID may not have

*It is true that strategies may take longer to teach in the ID population than in clients without ID. However, this does not mean that the client is incapable of learning to use fluency strategies.*

the words/vocabulary to do so. However, the behaviors they exhibit in response to their stuttering often demonstrate the manifestation of their frustration. Rather than saying, "I'm frustrated," the client may instead make a frustrated noise in response to stuttering blocks, use extra tension and/or other secondary behaviors to push through moments of blocks, and/or stop talking. They may avoid communicating in certain situations or engage in starting a phrase again to gain fluency (see Van Borsel & Tetnowski, 2007, for review). I have found that each client with ID is an individual when it comes to secondary behaviors. Although some exhibit moderate to severe tension, sometimes this tension is related to affective and cognitive components and sometimes not. I find you have to explore each client's feelings about getting stuck individually in a concrete way they can understand. Also keep in mind that all communication is behavior (Ylivisaker et al., 2007); therefore, getting information from significant others in the

*...you have to explore each client's feelings about getting stuck individually in a concrete way they can understand.*

client's life (parents, teachers, group home staff, etc.) will help you to tease out reactions to moments of stuttering. Because some of these clients may think more literally, you may want to think about affective and cognitive components as you might for a preschooler. That is, preschoolers may get frustrated during a difficult speech moment, but don't often hold on to this frustration beyond the moment. Therefore, the frustration is a situational issue rather than a general issue. At the end of this chapter is a checklist for further assessing affective and cognitive components in a client with ID. This checklist can be used to gather information on a client's reaction to disfluency (regardless of type of disfluency), their thoughts (cognitive components) and feelings (affective components) about their disfluency, and how long lasting these reactions are (i.e., are they talked about "beyond the moment" of struggle).

# WHAT EXECUTIVE FUNCTIONING ISSUES CAN I EXPECT IN THIS POPULATION?

Executive issues abound in ID. There is documentation that the frontal lobes of those with ID develop at a slow rate and may not fully develop (see Richer, Lachance, & Côté, 2016, for review). People with ID have also been noted to have less efficient executive functioning skills. Increased language impairment in people with ID is thought to coincide with decreased efficiency of executive functioning. (Richer et al., 2016).

People with autism spectrum disorder (ASD) are also diagnosed with or without ID. Even without ID, clients with ASD will still have difficulties with executive function (EF) related to attention to task, self-awareness, self-monitoring, response inhibition, goal setting, working memory, phonological encoding, retrieval, cognitive flexibility, problem solving, and/or task persistence. Typically, both those with autism with and without ID have these deficits, but it stands to reason, given increased EF deficits in ID, that these deficits would be more pronounced in someone with ASD who also has ID.

Given that those with ID tend to have delayed or disordered language across all language domains (Paul & Norbury, 2012), those with ID will find it difficult to not only self-regulate or problem solve but to use language to talk through a challenging situation. Therefore, we would expect a pattern of inflexibility coming from their inability to communicate and solve problems. This explains their need for a predictable environment. There is research to support that children with only a communication impairment are judged by peers as being less desirable to interact with socially than peers without a communication impairment (Gertner, Rice, & Hadley, 1994). This has strong ramifications for children with both issues with communication and cognitive flexibility. Over time, their difficulty with daily problem solving often leaves them isolated from social groups, where they would learn skills for problem solving. Soon the maladaptive behaviors of early childhood are reinforced, and the child stays "stuck" instead of growing in cognitive flexibility.

*Executive issues abound in ID.*

As clinicians, we must consider that we will have clients with ID on our caseloads who have gone through years of being "stuck." Their lack of flexibility and their difficulty with problem-solving skills will make working on their fluency challenging, but not impossible. In this chapter, I hope to present you with activities and ways of approaching tasks that help you to realize that successful learning and use of fluency strategies are possible.

The most common executive functioning issues that may get in the way of success in fluency therapy with someone with ID are likely to be self-awareness, self-monitoring/self-regulation, problem solving and inflexibility, task persistence, and working memory. Because these skills do not occur in a vacuum, but rather intermix in the course of therapy, I will describe how I've taken these potential weaknesses into account when planning therapy activities. Potential areas of difficulty in treatment and potential solutions are also listed in Table 6-1.

| TABLE 6-1 | | |
|---|---|---|
| **Executive Functioning Difficulties and Solutions** | | |
| *EXECUTIVE FUNCTIONING AREA* | *POTENTIAL BARRIERS TO SUCCESS DUE TO THESE WEAKNESSES* | *POTENTIAL SOLUTIONS TO OVERCOMING THE BARRIERS* |
| Self-awareness | • Inability to identify the problem as a whole<br>• Inability to identify disfluent moments to apply strategies | • Use a "coach"<br>• Client as "teacher" |
| Self-monitoring/self-regulation | • Inability to use resources to self-monitor and respond appropriately to speech disfluency | • Use a "coach"<br>• Client as teacher<br>• Goals attached to external rewards |
| Working memory | • Inability to recall what strategies are and/or what strategy to apply when<br>• Resistance to using pauses because worried will forget message | • Use synergistic approach<br>• Use code word that encompasses one type of speech to decrease cognitive load<br>• Working memory strategies and exercises |
| Inflexibility/problem solving | • Difficulty buying in to reasons for strategies vs. old, ineffective responses (shifting set)<br>• Difficulty with online problem solving to deal with moments of disfluency as they occur | • Client as teacher<br>• Goals for flexibility tied to external reinforcers<br>• Use a "coach"<br>• Present strategies in different ways to increase flexibility |
| Task persistence | • Giving up when a strategy does not come automatically and takes practice | • Break into smaller tasks and reward for smaller successes<br>• Increased modeling, decreased language |

# WHAT STRATEGIES CAN I USE FOR STUTTERING?

When treating any client with ID, I am sure that it is quite evident to clinicians that material must be made concrete. Pure fluency-shaping strategies such as continuous phonation require a high level of self-monitoring. Given that the ID population is not one that excels at self-monitoring, I have found stuttering modification strategies to be more helpful and realistic as a long-term way to manage this condition. This means that for mild repetitions that do not get in the way of the client attempting to communicate, there may not be much intervention at all. Applying a stuttering strategy like cancellation to a mild repetition has little long-term value. However, for clients with ID, it is likely that language difficulties contribute at least in part to their disfluency. Therefore, I have found many of my clients with ID who experience easy stuttered repetitions to be aided greatly by the use of pausing. Because stuttering in young children tends to occur more on utterances requiring more formulation (see Bloodstein & Bernstein Ratner, 2008, for review), it would stand to reason that pausing may help give them more time to formulate. For clients with stuttering blocks, teaching them to modify moments of blocks so that they can take back control and respond to them in an easier manner is beneficial. Clients can be taught to approach the start of sentences before a block occurs in an easier manner by using a preparatory set (also known as rainbow speech for more concrete learners, see also Chapter 5). However, given the difficulties with self-monitoring in ID, the more likely scenario is that a client will either learn to ease out of a block in the middle (pullout, Box 6-1; going to neutral, Activity 5-7) and change their approach to an easier start or use the easier start after the moment of block (cancellation, see Box 6-1). The longer the block, the more struggle the client feels, and the more likely they are to apply the strategy. Parents and clinicians may initially think it is important to cue for every block, regardless of length. However, for a child who is used to this block-ing pattern in their speech, it takes a lot more effort to think about applying the strategy than to con-tinue with their typical response to the disfluency. Because of the increased work needed to apply

*...those clients with ID have gone through years of being "stuck." Their lack of flexibility and their difficulty with problem-solving skills will make working on their fluency challenging, but not impossible.*

the strategy, they often don't see the functional value. Contrast this with a 12-year-old girl with ID whose case I consulted on. My colleague was conducting a language evaluation, and because this girl was stuttering with severe blocks, tension, and communication avoidance, my colleague asked if I would pop in and "take a look." After seeing that she was clearly giving up on communicating once she got caught in one of her frequent blocks, I attempted to teach her "rainbow speech." (see the end of this chapter and Chapter 5 for the activities and descriptions). Within minutes, she was applying this strategy to real blocks. Is this the type of response I always get when presenting the strategy to someone with ID and stuttering blocks? No. However, it is a fabulous illustration of how, when the gain is high enough, someone with ID can learn to apply the strategy. The actual strategy is not difficult for most clients to learn. What is difficult is the self-monitoring and problem solving necessary to discern good times to apply the strategies. That is why we need to build upon what is natural for these clients. That is, when a client feels, "I am very frustrated and now I see that there is an easier way to start," we will be able to maximize both their buy-in to how strategies can be helpful and their investment in work-ing to use them in real speech. At the end of this chapter are activities focusing on rainbow speech and pausing. Also included are activities that parents/caregivers can use on a daily basis to assist children with proactive practice of strategies.

Often I find that if a client just practices rainbow speech in a structured setting for a few minutes daily, the result goes further toward carryover than might initially be suspected. In my experience, if the client is doing this practice every day as a routine, it is more likely that they will apply strategies to real moments of stuttering blocks. Additionally, I talk with clients and their loved ones about thinking of this daily practice as a way to keep overall disfluency down. Although most structured therapy pro-grams require daily practice, the specific contribution that daily practice makes to long-term fluency is unknown. Anecdotally, I do find that clients who engage in this practice show reduction in disfluency. The reduction may be because the client is more aware of fluency strategies. It may be because they are approaching blocks in an effective rather than ineffective manner and/or they are breaking the cycle of responding to stuttering with tension and avoidance. It may be because the consistent practice helps parents remain cognizant of encouraging communication at all times in their child who stutters, or because consistent practice establishes a valuable low-communication-stress routine between the care-giver and client (see Swift et al., 2016, for review). It may be something completely different than any of these reasons. Until we know the specific reason, we can say that daily practice is something consistent parents can do that seems to be beneficial overall.

# WHAT STRATEGIES CAN I USE FOR CLUTTERING?

For cluttering treatment with the ID population, many of my clients respond best to finding the one strategy that provides the most "bang for the buck." As mentioned, self-monitoring is difficult

| Box 6-1 | | |
| --- | --- | --- |
| **Stuttering Strategies** | | |
| *TYPE* | *DEFINITION* | *EXAMPLES* |
| Fluency shaping | Used proactively throughout all speech; goal is to use strategies to avoid stuttering. | • Continuous phonation* (keeping voicing going between words; connecting end of one word to beginning of next word) |
| Stuttering modification (Van Riper, 1973) | Used proactively (preparatory set) and mostly reactively in response to a moment of stuttering; goal is to manage moments of stuttering without applying strategies throughout all speech. | • Preparatory set (gentle stretch of first vowel in word before a moment of stuttering; e.g., moooomy)<br>• Pullout (gentle slide out when in the middle of a moment of stuttering by stretching vowel; e.g., mo—oooomy)<br>• Cancellation (preparatory set applied after a moment of stuttering to take back control) |

*Continuous phonation

**What you do:** The idea of continuous phonation is to keep your voicing from your vocal cords constantly going while you talk.

**How you do it:** Try to connect all of your words as you talk. Think about connecting the end of one word to the beginning of the next word. After a long phrase or sentence, when you have a natural pause in speech, start your next phrase or sentence with continuous phonation, connecting all of the words.

**Note**: When first using this strategy, your voice will sound more monotone. This will lessen as you get faster with connecting the words.

in clients with ID. Our best bet is to take advantage of the synergistic principle, whereby treating one area transfers to improvements in other areas (Myers & Bradley, 1992). By following this principle, we will require the smallest cognitive load for our clients to use strategies, thereby giving them the best chance for success (Scaler Scott & Ward, 2013). In terms of speech intelligibility for those who clutter, the most effective strategy I have found to help clients use a rate that is more in sync with what their motor system can handle is increasing natural pausing in speech. For some clients, this may be enough to make an overall positive impact upon speech intelligibility. If the client also stutters (see previous section), pausing may also provide the benefit of decreasing easy repetitions, as it may provide more time for formulation of thoughts. Be sure that your clients are pausing for at least the amount of time it takes them to say "one" in their heads, as often without this cue, I find their pauses are too short to be discernible and to make a significant difference to their listener(s) and to their intelligibility.

For some clients, pausing is not enough. Some of my clients with cluttering will pause but will speed through their words between the pauses. When this happens, there is some improvement in overall intelligibility, but not enough to be considered completely successful. Therefore, I next teach the idea of emphasizing all sounds and syllables in words. I especially teach clients that focusing on emphasizing ending sounds is most helpful to the listener. We talk about emphasis in a way that sounds natural to the listener. Although the extra emphasis may feel unnatural to your clients at first, keep in mind that clients with excessive over-coarticulation or "mushy speech" come to you using too little emphasis. Therefore, increased emphasis is likely to sound clear rather than unnatural to their listeners. For some clients, I have found that when they focus on emphasizing only, it results in a slower rate of speech (but in a natural way), therefore having a positive impact upon overall intelligibility. For other clients, they may need to pause and emphasize sounds. Given that your clients with ID will be concrete, you may want to make up one code word that implies both pausing and emphasizing. Of course, this code word has to be meaningful to your client. For example, one client I worked with who had ID loved the sound of the voice of the Smart Board used in his classroom. The voice was slower than his and very emphasized, as it was digitized. Both aspects (slow and emphasized) helped him to focus on

> *...we will require the smallest cognitive load for our clients to use strategies, thereby giving them the best chance for success (Scaler Scott & Ward, 2013)*

pausing and emphasizing. His teachers and I decided that the cue, "Talk like the Smart Board" was the best cue to give him for speech clarity. Of course, we did not want him to use a digitized-sounding voice whenever he spoke, as this would sound quite artificial and cause more pragmatic problems. His voice sounded artificial in the beginning, then we shaped it to telling him to sound like a newer Smart Board, one that sounded more like a human and less like a robot. With lots of modeling and practice, he got it! At the end of this chapter are specific exercises to teach pausing and emphasizing.

Cues and prompts are very important to the client with ID; however, if they are not looking at the person cueing or prompting them, then the cues are of little value. Often with clients without ID, I teach them to be a "detective" and while they are speaking with someone to carefully examine the listener's face for signs that they may not be understanding (Scaler Scott & Ward, 2013). As soon as they see signs of confusion, that is their cue to change the way they are speaking, whether that be to increase pauses, emphasize sounds, or whatever is found to make them the most clear. For clients who are more concrete, those around them can be taught to use a confused face the client can look out for. However, it should be kept in mind that clients either will not be comfortable with consistent eye contact or may not engage in it due to the conversational exchange (e.g., parent in front of moving car, child in back). Therefore, the child can also be taught to be a detective by listening for signs of confusion. The client listens for a code word that will help them know that their listener is not understanding. It should be a simple term, like "huh?" or "what?" or "again?" Just as with responding to the confused face, the client responds to the confused voice by making their statement again, but modifying it to be clearer (by, for example, increasing pausing and/or emphasizing). Often my clients who are more concrete need much reinforcement and practice with changing how they respond when communication breaks down. They need a great deal of practice responding to communication breakdowns by implementing strategies rather than by just repeating what they said in the same manner.

Another strategy I have found works very well with more concrete clients is the idea of putting them in the role of "teacher" (Gottwald & Dietrich, 2002). I'm sure you've heard the concept that if you can teach something, you are demonstrating that you truly understand it (Shulman, 1986). If we apply this principle to our concrete clients, we can put them in the role of "teacher." We can use mushy speech and have them cue us (e.g., "Use pausing," "Make your sounds clear," etc.). During such practice, respond to the client's cues with an appropriate response only sometimes. When you respond appropriately, praise the client for being such a good teacher and helping you speak clearly. Several times, do not respond appropriately so that you need to be cued again by the client. Having the client learn to cue us, praise us, and give us feedback when we need to try again helps familiarize them with the process for when the roles are reversed. Additionally, during their "teaching" the client can start listening to the responses of others (typically those of the clinician and/or caregiver), judging whether or not each response is accurate. The long-term goal of judging the correctness of others' responses is to help clients tune in to their own speech. Included at the end of this chapter is a sample activity for putting the child in the role of teacher.

# WHAT TO DO ABOUT ATYPICAL STUTTERING

I am often asked these questions, and when working with someone with ID and trying to balance priorities, I think the questions are valid. There are some clients, whether diagnosed with ID or not, who are aware of their atypical disfluencies and experience negative feelings and attitudes in response to them. These are definitely cases where the disfluencies should be addressed. If a client feels badly about the disfluencies and this results in them communicating less, then there is negative impact upon class or work participation and/or participation in social interaction. In these clients, treatment of atypical disfluency needs to be addressed. In clients who are unaware of their disfluency and for whom there is no negative impact upon their attempts at communication, atypical disfluency might be set aside until the timing is more appropriate to address.

Recent work we are conducting (Scaler Scott et al., in preparation) indicates that some clients will place a pause before a repetition at the end of the word and some will not. Many clients use both forms of disfluency. We do not yet know what differentiates these two types of disfluency, but speculate that the pauses may be more related to an internal distraction as described later, and the form without pauses may be related more to a motoric behavior. Continued research is needed in this area.

For a client whom the clinician deems needs to address their atypical disfluency, the only published treatment research involves two case studies focused upon identification and correction of disfluencies (Sisskin & Wasilus, 2014; Van Borsel, Geirneart, & Van Coster, 2005). One of these two cases also focused upon use of phrasing strategies (Van Borsel et al., 2005). Having worked with some students who are quite sensitive to their atypical disfluency and coming from the mind-set that the disfluency is not something within the client's control, I prefer to focus on what seems to be possible underlying factors contributing to their disfluency. Why and how are they using the disfluency? (although it may not be a conscious decision to do so; Scaler Scott & Sisskin, 2007; Sisskin & Scaler Scott, 2007). We do not consciously choose to use filler words such as "um" or "uh" to signal we are thinking of a word or thought, but we do so nonetheless (Clark & Fox Tree, 2002). Considering the idea that those with atypical disfluency may be using their disfluency in a similar manner allows us to see atypical disfluency as a sign of formulation trouble. From there we can assess what the trouble may be. Is it because the client is having trouble coming up with the next word? The next thought? Do they not want to insert a pause because they are afraid someone else will take

*There are some clients, whether diagnosed with ID or not, who are aware of their atypical disfluencies and experience negative feelings and attitudes in response to them.*

the floor and they will forget their point (a common complaint of my clients with atypical disfluencies)? Depending on the answers to these questions, the clinician can address the relevant areas: word retrieval, language organization, working memory, etc. In preliminary testing of a small sample of school-aged children with WFDs (Scaler Scott, et al., in preparation), these were the three areas most negatively affected in testing. For each child, although they may have presented with difficulties in each of these areas, the proportion of difficulty within each area was not the same. Therefore, by conducting testing and creating a profile of their client with atypical disfluency, the clinician can figure out the priorities for treatment. It should be kept in mind that at times this treatment has correlated with a decrease in or elimination of WFDs, but that complete elimination is not always certain. However, if the clinician is focusing upon aspects of language that need to be treated anyway, this is something that can benefit the client, regardless of its impact upon atypical disfluencies. This may represent the best solution until further research data on clinical efficacy are available. Tables 6-2 through 6-4 guide the clinician through testing the potential contributing factors to atypical disfluencies and planning appropriate intervention based upon the results of testing. An outline of a sample lesson for addressing the atypical disfluencies is also included.

| TABLE 6-2 | | |
|---|---|---|
| **Identifying Areas to Treat in Atypical Disfluencies** | | |
| *SUSPECTED CONTRIBUTOR TO DISFLUENCY* | *WAYS TO TEST THIS* | *ACTIVITIES TO INTERVENE IN THESE AREAS* |
| Word retrieval | Standardized tests of vocabulary and word finding: Peabody Picture Vocabulary Test, Fourth Edition (PPTVT-4); Expressive Vocabulary Test, Second Edition (EVT-2); Test of Word Finding; Word Associations subtest of the Clinical Evaluation of Language Fundamentals, Fourth Edition (CELF-4) | • Activities involving antonyms, synonyms, categorization (foundation level)<br>• Activities involving descriptions and definitions<br>• Use of visual organizers for verbal narratives |
| Language organization | Sentence Assembly and Recalling Sentences subtests of CELF-5; Word Associations subtest of the CELF-4; Test of Narrative Language, Second Edition (TNL-2); samples in monologue and expository discourse | • Use of visual organizers for verbal narratives |
| Working memory | Understanding Spoken Paragraphs subtest of the CELF-5; Comprehensive Test of Phonological Processing, Second Edition (CTOPP-2): Memory for Digits and Nonword Repetition subtests; Test of Auditory Processing Skills, Third Edition (TAPS-3) | • Use of visualization strategies |

# SAMPLE TEST SCORES AND LESSON PLAN FOR ATYPICAL DISFLUENCIES

Client is a 9-year, 8-month-old male. He was diagnosed with and being treated for central auditory processing disorder and social pragmatic difficulties via speech therapy at his school. His mother noticed WFDs. As shown in Table 6-3, he scored within the average range on most tests except two subtests focusing on memory. Qualitatively, he also demonstrated some inaccurate use of irregular past-tense verbs. He showed increased WFDs as formulation demands increased, such as during story retell tasks and when attempting to make multiple sentences out of given words on the Sentence Assembly subtest of the CELF-5. It was thought that he might benefit from extra time to formulate, which could be facilitated by using visual organizers and increasing his pausing. However, given that he has difficulty holding things in his memory, he needs to be taught strategies to assist with this so that he doesn't lose the information while pausing. It was also felt that working on complex grammatical forms and irregular past-tense verbs might increase efficiency of formulation. Therefore, the plan for this client, as outlined in Table 6-4, was to introduce visualization to compensate for difficulties with memory, pausing to compensate for difficulties with formulation, and categorization to work on the foundation level skill of language organization. Ultimately, the plan for this client is to be able to hold onto language information while formulating ideas in conversation and story telling.

| TABLE 6-3 | | |
|---|---|---|
| **Sample Test Scores for Atypical Disfluencies** | | |
| *TEST* | *NORMS* | *CLIENT* |
| *Peabody Picture Vocabulary Test 4 (PPVT-4)* | Standard Score: 100 + or − 15 <br> Percentile Rank: 50 + or − 25 | Standard Score: 95 <br> Percentile Rank: 37 |
| *Expressive Vocabulary Test 2 (EVT-2)* | Standard Score: 100 + or − 15 <br> Percentile Rank: 50 + or − 25 | Standard Score: 96 <br> Percentile Rank: 39 |
| *Test of Auditory Processing Skills (TAPS-3):* <br> *Word Memory* | Scaled Score: 10 + or − 3 <br> Percentile Rank: 50 = or − 25 | Scaled Score: 8 <br> Percentile Rank: 25 |
| *Test of Auditory Processing Skills (TAPS-3):* <br> *Sentence Memory* | Scaled Score: 10 + or − 3 <br> Percentile Rank: 50 = or − 25 | Scaled Score: 3 <br> Percentile Rank: 1 |
| *Comprehensive Test of Phonological Processing 2 (CTOPP-2):* <br> *Memory for Digits* | Scaled Score: 10 + or − 3 <br> Percentile Rank: 50 = or − 25 | Scaled Score: 8 <br> Percentile Rank: 25 |
| *Comprehensive Test of Phonological Processing 2 (CTOPP-2):* <br> *Nonword Repetition* | Scaled Score: 10 + or − 3 <br> Percentile Rank: 50 = or − 25 | Scaled Score: 5 <br> Percentile Rank: 5 |
| *Clinical Evaluation of Language Fundamentals (CELF-4):* <br> *Recalling Sentences* | Scaled Score: 10 + or − 3 <br> Percentile Rank: 50 = or − 25 | Scaled Score: 9 <br> Percentile Rank: 37 |
| *Clinical Evaluation of Language Fundamentals (CELF-5):* <br> *Sentence Assembly* | Scaled Score: 10 + or − 3 <br> Percentile Rank: 50 = or − 25 | Scaled Score: 9 <br> Percentile Rank: 37 |
| *Clinical Evaluation of Language Fundamentals (CELF-4):* <br> *Understanding Spoken Paragraphs* | Scaled Score: 10 + or − 3 <br> Percentile Rank: 50 = or − 25 | Scaled Score: 8 <br> Percentile Rank: 25 |
| *Clinical Evaluation of Language Fundamentals (CELF-3):* <br> *Word Associations* | Standard Score: 100 + or − 15 <br> Percentile Rank: 50 + or − 25 | Standard Score: 8 <br> Percentile Rank: 25 |

| TABLE 6-4 | | | | |
|-----------|---|---|---|---|
| **Example of Lesson Plan Based Upon Test Scores and Potential Contributors to Atypical Disfluencies** | | | | |
| *WEEK* | *SKILL* | *ACTIVITY* | *RATIONALE* | *HOME ACTIVITY* |
| 1 | Introduction to visualizing | Discuss what it means to imagine or visualize | To provide background | Describe what you picture while reading stories |
| | | Describe object or picture | To build visualization skill | |
| | Introduction to pausing | In Crazy 8s (I am putting down//a 6 of hearts) | To provide more time for formulation | Practice Crazy 8s or other game with pausing |
| | Introduction to categories and organizing | Subcategories | To improve verbal organization | Play subcategory/category games in car |

# ACTIVITY 6-1:
## CAREGIVER QUESTIONNAIRE

1. When my child has trouble with fluency, their reaction is to (please circle all that apply):
   - Cry
   - Express frustration
   - Yell
   - Stop talking
   - Say "forget it"
   - No reaction
   - Other reaction to disfluency:


2. My child talks about their speech being difficult at times when they are not having trouble:
   ☐ Yes      ☐ No


3. Things my child says about their speech WHILE they are having trouble:




4. Things my child says about their speech while they are NOT having trouble:

# ACTIVITY 6-2: RAINBOW SPEECH

Rainbow speech is a child-friendly name for preparatory set. This kind of speech often makes it easier to start a word, as many who stutter have difficulty getting the sounds started. Rainbow speech changes the timing and tension of speech to make getting started easier. The timing is changed by gently prolonging the first vowel in the word. The tension is changed by gently stretching the vowel.

*Materials needed*: Paper and crayons, markers, or colored pencils

## Presenting the Concept

**Clinician**: Do you know what a rainbow is? They have lots of pretty colors in them. Let's pick out a few colors and we will make a rainbow together.

**Clinician**: I will draw the first part so I can show you how we do it in speech. What color should I use first?

**Clinician**: Okay, you chose red. I will use red first. Listen to how I say the word "red" while I draw. Reeed. (gentle stretch on "e" sound; clinician starts saying the word as soon as she or he starts drawing and doesn't end the word until the end of the arc is reached). In this way, the clinician is modeling a long stretch. Upon presentation in this manner, the clinician wants to exaggerate the model of the stretched vowel for the child. This is because in real situations the child will tend to shorten the vowel. Therefore, you don't want the stretched vowel to start short and then in real life be nonexistent.

**Clinician**: Now you try. See if you can trace my red line and say "reeeed." Cues: Make sure you keep saying the word until you get to the end of the rainbow.

**Clinician**: Good, you got red. Now let's pick another color to try. I'll go first. "yeeeellow". Now you try. Repeat as often as child needs to get the concept of how to gently stretch the vowel. Once the child seems to understand this concept, they can move to "teaching" you.

**Clinician**: You're so good at this! I'll bet you can teach me/mom/dad (any significant other who may be present for the session). Can you pick a new color and show us?

**Client**: Green (draws rainbow quickly and says "green" quickly).

**Clinician**: Remember the word has to get stretched out like this, "greeeen." And we have to keep stretching it until we get to the end of the rainbow, like this, "greeen."

After teaching the concept of what rainbow speech is, the idea is that the child will learn to use it to start speech in an easier manner. Following are some ideas that will help facilitate this process. Do keep in mind that if a child is really struggling to get sounds out and you teach them an easier way to do so, they are likely to adopt the rainbow speech on their own with little intervention on your part. I have found this to be the case with some students with ID. All I have to do is tell them it's an easier way to start their speech, and they are off and running. With others they need more help in connecting that this strategy is what we use when we are really stuck. Here are some ideas to help the child make the connection between use of the strategy and getting stuck.

## Daily Practice With Rainbow Speech

Following are ideas to practice rainbow speech proactively daily. These practice sessions are meant to be short. The rationale behind them is to 1) help keep strategies in the forefront of a client's mind for when they need to use them during real moments of stuttering and 2) gain structured practice with using the strategy before applying it to real situations. In the next section are ideas for daily quick practice of rainbow speech. I tell my clients that they will do about 5 minutes (about 10 sentences) of daily practice with rainbow speech. Caregivers and clients are taught that this is their daily practice to make sure they keep their speech healthy.

# ACTIVITY 6-3:
## IDEAS FOR RAINBOW SPEECH GAMES

## *Daily Practice With Rainbow Speech*

Following are ideas to practice rainbow speech proactively daily. These practice sessions are meant to be short. The rationale behind them is to 1) help keep strategies in the forefront of a client's mind for when they need to use them during real moments of stuttering and 2) gain structured practice with using the strategy before applying it to real situations. In the next section are ideas for daily quick practice of rainbow speech. I tell my clients that they will do about 5 minutes (about 10 sentences) of daily practice with rainbow speech. Caregivers and clients are taught that this is their daily practice to make sure they keep their speech healthy.

### Quick Games

- Count on your fingers to 10
- Name objects in room (IIII see a chair; Here is a coooouch)
- Name objects while riding in car (Theeeere is a stop sign)
- Name objects on one page of a book
- Color a rainbow
- Say a magic spell to make Mommy or Daddy dance or sing:

  Aaabracadabra

  IIII want to see Mommy sing

  Sheee will sing a song

  IIIt will be a Christmas song

  Wheeen I say go

  Sheee will sing it

  Sheee will sing "Jingle Bells"

  Aaand she will dance

  Aaare you ready Mommy?

  Gooo ahead and sing

### Slower Games

- Eye Spy (give clues and try to guess)
  - IIII spy with my little eye
  - Sooomething red
  - IIIIt is big
- Surprise stretch while reading a book—whoever does the most wins
  - Child and caregiver take turns stretching a word at random times
  - e.g., "Heeere is a dog"

## Troubleshooting Tips for Rainbow Speech

Sometimes when a client tries to stretch out the first vowel, they become stuck on the first consonant of the word and cannot move forward. In these cases, it is best to teach the concept of light touch of the articulators (see also activities in Chapter 5). In light contact or touch, the client touches the articulators together gently. Often when a child adjusts and touches their articulators gently, they are able to move forward with stretching the vowel sound for rainbow speech. Sometimes, however, the child still becomes locked on the consonant sound. That is, they may return to try the consonant sound again, but become stuck again. If this is the case, the client can try to say the consonant sound while blowing a little air out to get the sound moving. So, for example, they might blow some air out about the same time they are gently trying to touch their top teeth to their bottom lip when saying the word "ffff-fuuuun." It is important to only use this technique when needed and to blow the air concurrently with producing the sound. In this way, the client is not establishing a new pattern of first attempting to blow air (in an obvious and disruptive manner) as a "trick" to get words out.

# ACTIVITY 6-4:
## CHILD AS TEACHER

Clinician and child play any age-appropriate game. I usually use things like Eye Spy or guessing objects that I pull out of a bag, etc. As I am taking my turn in the game, I simulate blocking on a word. I hold the block and say to the child, "My word is stuck. Can you help me?" (Note: Often I find that the client doesn't "catch on" that I am actually not stuck when I am asking for help.) Next I say, "What should I do?" Often the child does not know, so I say, "Tell me, use rainbow speech, Miss Kathy." The child repeats what I say (or if a caregiver or other person is in the session, they can cue me first as a model). I use rainbow speech and then say, "Wow, that made speech so easy. My word was stuck. That helped it come out. Thanks for helping me." I do this as much as needed for the child to get the concept of how to help me. If the child is able to "teach" me what to do, this means they will better know what a parent or other adult is going for when they cue them to use rainbow speech. Sometimes when they cue me I will deliberately keep pushing the word out, and say, "Is this rainbow speech?" When the child says "no," I will respond, "You have to show me. I need help learning it." In this way the client is learning what to do (use rainbow speech) and what not to do (don't push or fight against word).

The child can also learn to "teach" the clinician how to pause to help others understand their speech (such as in cluttering) or to pause for silent thinking (such as in atypical disfluency).

# ACTIVITY 6-5:
## ADULT CUE IN REAL MOMENTS

After the client has gotten the concept of how rainbow speech makes talking easier, you can cue them to use rainbow speech in moments when they are stuck. You can practice this in sessions with the client and teach parents/caregivers/teachers to also implement this at home. When the client is stuck in a block and you know what word they are trying to say, you gently cue them to use rainbow speech by modeling: "Try (word said with rainbow speech)." For example, if you know they are trying to say "mom," you say, "Try moooom." When they follow your model, you praise their effort by saying something like, "You really used your rainbow speech. That made your word come out easier." What is important to note is that if a client is really stuck and you are cueing them in a gentle manner, it is okay to interrupt their block to help coach them through a strategy. This is important to stress as you may at first find it counterintuitive to interrupt a child in the middle of a stutter. However, if you are gently providing "online coaching" in this manner, it is the best way for clients to learn when to apply strategies to real moments. If the client has a mild block that they get through quickly, this type of online coaching might not be as effective. However, sometimes it is difficult to catch a block right at the moment it is occurring. If a client has struggled through a word, you could then say, "Try mooom." This would be a form of cancellation that would help the client connect strategy use to being stuck. It is always best to catch the stutter in the middle, but not always possible. First we would aim to catch it in the middle, next right after the stutter. If the child has moved on several words, you wouldn't want to cue them at that time, as that moment is likely too far removed from the moment of stuttering for them to connect the block to the strategy.

In a similar manner, adults can cue for increased pausing to help with cluttering and/or atypical disfluency. Work out a signal with your child/student that is recognizable to them to shift to pausing.

# ACTIVITY 6-6:
# MODELING CONJUNCTIONS IN REAL LIFE

Conjunctions are words that connect one idea in a sentence to another. Examples of conjunctions are: and, but, so, except, and because. As young children are building more complex sentences, they begin to use conjunctions more and more. As more complex language begins to develop, preschoolers tend to say one complex sentence as two different sentences (e.g., "You have to get gas in the car" (pause while playing) "Because you need gas"). Later, they use conjunctions in the middle of sentences, as older children and adults do (e.g., "I don't want to go to bed because I am not tired").

For some preschoolers, increased complexity of language may increase disfluency. Teaching a child silent thinking (through your own modeling) can help until complex language becomes more stable. The following are some ways you can do this:

1. Model use of complex sentences with silent thinking as part of everyday conversation with your child. Examples:
   - "I don't think we can go outside **because** (silent thinking) it's raining."
   - "Let's get on your coat **so** (silent thinking) we can go outside."
   - "You have to clean up all the toys (silent thinking) **except** the puzzle."
   - "You ate most of your dinner **but** (silent thinking) you need to eat your beans."
   - "We are going to the store **and** (silent thinking) then we are going to the party."

2. In conversation, you can also elicit these types of sentences from your child by modeling silent thinking with choices.
   - Example 1:
     **Child**: "I want to go outside."
     **Adult**: "Do you want to go outside **so** (silent thinking) you can play in the snow (pause) or do you want to go outside (silent thinking) **so** you can play with the balls?"
   - Example 2:
     **Child**: "I want that cereal."
     **Adult**: "Do you want that cereal **because** (silent thinking) it tastes better (pause) or do you want that cereal (silent thinking) **because** you like the colors?"

Do this in moderation and don't worry if your child doesn't respond exactly as you model.

If you hear spontaneous use of silent thinking, provide verbal praise, such as, "You used silent thinking! That helps us think of how to say something. Grown-ups use it too."

**Note**: You can pause before or after the conjunction, whatever feels more natural to you. Some like to pause after the conjunction because usually what comes next may require some time to formulate. Others like to pause after the conjunction because it lets the listener know there is more information coming. There is no hard-and-fast rule; the pause place should just feel relatively natural to you.

**Also**: If a client tries to jump in while you are pausing, gently stop them and say, "I'm still talking, I need a minute to think." This will teach them that silent pause time is for the speaker to gather thoughts, and their job is to wait patiently.

**Sometimes**: Caregivers are concerned that their child will ask, "Why are you talking so slowly?" or "Why are you waiting?" if they have not encountered the caregiver doing this before. I have found that children tend to ask about this about 10% of the time. To be prepared for those questions, I tell caregivers they can respond by saying, "We are trying to do things a little more slowly in this house. So if we need more time to think, we are not rushing through; we are just taking the time we need."

**Remember**: This advice does not mean to tell a child to slow down and/or think about what they want to say, as neither are fluency-enhancing statements. It is simply to help them build in pause time that they may need as language is developing.

# ACTIVITY 6-7:
# LOOKING FOR THE CONFUSED FACE—HUH? WHAT?

Teach the client to look for confusion on other's faces so they can correct that confusion by using a strategy to clear up their speech.

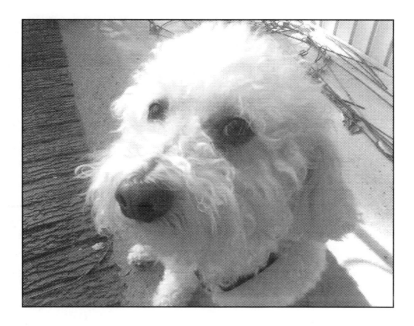

# ACTIVITY 6-8:
# PAUSING (FOR CLUTTERING OR ATYPICAL DISFLUENCY)

Teach the client to pause at commas and periods while reading. If your client is not a reader, teach them to retell a story with pictures, pausing in natural places.

## *Reader Story*

Once there was a boy//who liked to play//with his dog//. His dog had white fur//with brown patches on it//. The dog's name//was Lucky//. Lucky was a very smart dog//and he liked to jump//up and down// on his back legs//. He did this a lot//when he wanted a treat.

**Note**: For nonreader story, use a series of pictures that tell a story. Adult tells it and child practices telling it back, with focus on pausing.

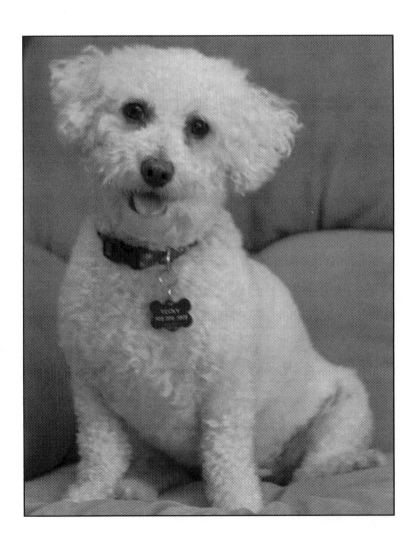

# ACTIVITY 6-9:
## EMPHASIS FOR UNCLEAR SPEECH

Teach clients whose speech is unclear to emphasize word endings. To make this concept more concrete, you might not say "emphasize" but rather say something like, "Say the sounds stronger at the end." For your clients who are readers, you can use a book and underline word endings. For your non-reader clients, you can model how to stress ending sounds via picture or object naming. Just remember that for modeling you may want to exaggerate at first, as a child is likely to lessen the model in real-life situations. However, you know your client best. If you feel over-exaggeration will lead to them emphasizing unnaturally long term, then do not over-exaggerate. That is completely an individual call based upon the client. Following is an example of a picture and stimulus sentence:

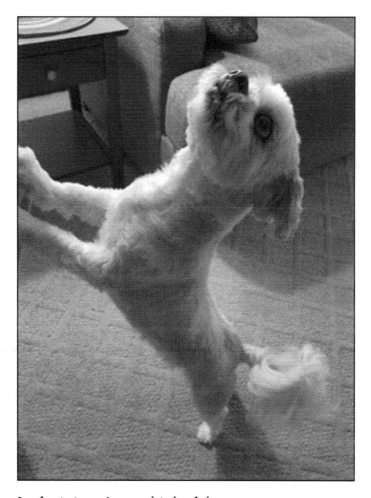

Lu**ck**y is jump**ing** on his ba**ck** le**gs**.

# ACTIVITY 6-10:
# BINGO BOARD

This activity helps with carryover of tasks. The client takes home a bingo board with spaces filled in for goals they are working on. As they complete a task at home, they fill in the appropriate square (color it in, place stickers on it, etc.). The goal is to bring back a completed full card for a prize. You can change this board (see next page) to target goals related to stuttering and/or cluttering and/or atypical stuttering, depending on the client's needs. What follows is an example of a board for a client with ID, stuttering, and cluttering.

| B | I | N | G | O |
|---|---|---|---|---|
| clear request | clear request | clear speech | clear speech | clear speech |
| rainbow speech | clear reading | rainbow speech | clear speech | emphasize sounds |
| clear request | rainbow speech | clear conversation | pause | clear request |
| rainbow speech | rainbow speech | pause | emphasize sounds | clear reading |
| pause | clear request | clear request | clear request | pause |

| B | I | N | G | O |
|---|---|---|---|---|
|   |   |   |   |   |
|   |   |   |   |   |
|   |   |   |   |   |
|   |   |   |   |   |
|   |   |   |   |   |

# CHAPTER 7

# LEARNING DISABILITIES, AUDITORY PROCESSING, AND LANGUAGE DISORDERS

## DELINEATION OF TERMS

When we are talking about the disorder categories in this chapter, it is important to distinguish between them. The category of learning disability in the United States is diagnosed when a student, despite average to above-average intelligence quotient (IQ), has difficulty with academic performance due to difficulties in how the brain receives and processes information. Problems may be identified in areas such as reading, writing, mathematics, listening, spelling, and some related movement disorders (National Center for Learning Disabilities, 2013). The National Center for Learning Disabilities (NCLD, 2013) considers the aforementioned academic disability areas to be central to learning disorders and the following difficulties to be "associated disorders," which may coexist with a learning disability: dyspraxia, executive function disorders, attention deficit hyperactivity disorder (ADHD), auditory processing disorder, and visual processing disorder. Disorder categories such as ADHD and visual processing disorder are not language-based. It should be noted that in some parts of the world , learning disabilities equate to intellectual disability, where IQ scores are below average. Recall that intellectual disability is covered in the previous chapter of this book.

For the purposes of this chapter, when we speak of learning disabilities, we will include both those difficulties considered by the NCLD as central to a diagnosis of learning disability and those associated with the diagnosis. We will be referring to academic challenges that are based in areas serviced by the speech-language clinician. Therefore, an auditory processing disorder, which negatively affects how a person's brain takes in and understands the language they hear, has a negative impact upon classroom performance (such as following directions and reading comprehension), and is based in language. Literacy disorders (related to difficulties with reading, writing, and/or spelling) are often the expression of an underlying language disorder. This chapter will deal with learning disabilities and their associated symptoms based in language. Attention deficit disorder will be dealt with in a separate chapter.

Those with learning disorders have the same ability to learn (based upon IQ being average to above average) as those without learning disorders. The difference with someone with a learning disorder is that they may need information to be presented differently than someone without a learning disorder.

Scaler Scott, K.
*Fluency Plus: Managing Fluency Disorders in*
*Individuals With Multiple Diagnoses (pp 109-130).*
© 2018 Taylor & Francis Group.

Therefore, there are some who advocate for the term *learning difference* rather than *learning disorder*. The terms learning disorder, learning disability, and learning difference will be used synonymously in this chapter and book.

# WHAT FLUENCY DISORDERS ARE COMMONLY FOUND IN THIS POPULATION?

I have worked with numerous children with language-based learning differences (LLDs) in school, outpatient hospital, and private settings. Within the population of LLD, I have seen many cases of concomitant cluttering. The literature at one time described cluttering as a complex syndrome of learning disabilities (Tiger, Irvine, & Reis, 1980). Auditory processing difficulties and difficulties with attention to auditory tasks have been found in those with cluttering (Blood, Blood, & Tellis, 1997, 1999, 2000). Deceased efficiency in processing syntactical forms has been found in children (Usler & Weber-Fox, 2015) and adults (see Usler & Weber-Fox, 2015, for review) who stutter. It is also known that disfluency in general (stuttering and non-stuttering) is seen more in clients with overt language disorders and/or in clients with subtle language disorders that are not identified on testing (see Bloodstein & Bernstein Ratner, 2008, for review). Word-final disfluencies have been identified in children with literacy disorders (Sutkowski, Tokach, & Scaler Scott, 2015), and attention disorders (Scaler Scott, Grossman, Abendroth, Tetnowski, & Damico, 2007). When the clinician is evaluating a client with any type of learning disability, it is warranted that they observe, test for, and ask about symptoms related to stuttering, cluttering, atypical disfluency, and excessive normal disfluency.

> *Those with learning disorders have the same ability to learn (based upon IQ being average to above average) as those without learning disorders.*

# MYTHS AND FACTS ABOUT FLUENCY DISORDERS IN INDIVIDUALS WITH LEARNING DIFFERENCES

The first myth about clients with learning disorders is that many of them are just not motivated. It is important to note that after years of school failure, clients may have developed difficulties with self-regulation of behavior during assignments they find challenging, such as language-based assignments. For some with learning disabilities, it is difficult to distinguish between what executive functioning (EF) issues are neurologically based and what issues are the result of response to academic failure. The significant impact academic failure has on a child's response to school and assignments should never be underestimated, especially in older school-aged children. Academic failure can lead to a host of issues affecting academic performance, such as depression and/or anxiety (see Fisher, Allen, & Kose, 1996, for review). The impact of academic failure may only be seen if the clinician is working on a language-based task, but might also be seen for all tasks presented in general. The clinician is encouraged to work closely with a counselor or therapist to assist the client in coping with these issues to ensure the best performance possible in speech-language sessions.

There is a parallel between school failure and failure of fluency therapy. Some children have experienced fluency therapy that has been less than helpful because their clinician was not trained in effective approaches. This may also be the case for someone with a severe reading disability. I have worked with numerous students with dyslexia who have made it to high school and tried multiple approaches, none of which helped them to significantly progress in reading. It is no wonder these students become less and less motivated to try as the years go on. If you as a clinician are "inheriting" a client who is frustrated with previous approaches to their treatment, whether it be for fluency or learning differences or both, you are likely to encounter some skepticism from your client. I have found the best way to overcome this is to talk with your client early on about what they have done in previous therapy and what they have and have not found helpful. Such a discussion aids the clinician in better understanding the techniques they may not want to repeat with their client. That being

*After years of school failure, clients may have developed difficulties with self-regulation of behavior during assignments they find challenging, such as language-based assignments.*

said, keep in mind that sometimes a presented technique may have been the right one for a given client, but it wasn't presented in the correct manner, or the client and/or caregiver misunderstood its purpose or how to effectively execute the technique. It also could have simply been that the technique was presented at a time when the client was not ready for it. If you suspect that any of these scenarios are the case, do not try and convince your client about the merit of a given strategy. Instead, talk with them about the rationale behind any techniques you present and the efficacy data for them. Acknowledge that they may not have found these techniques helpful in the past, explain why that might have been, and explain how you and your client will use the strategy differently together. Most importantly, emphasize to clients and caregivers that they need to feel free to ask questions about anything you do at any time and that they need to be open if they don't understand a given technique and/or don't think it is working for them. Tell them that it is a waste of everyone's time for them to politely say they will follow a strategy you present when they have no intention of doing so. Finally, tell caregivers that you want to hear any criticism the client has, as the client may be more willing to give that feedback to a parent or spouse than to the clinician.

One last myth that must be dealt with relates to the diagnosis of dyslexia. When someone has difficulty sounding out words to read and/or spell, they may be diagnosed with dyslexia. Dyslexia is considered a language-based learning disability because someone with dyslexia has key issues with associating letters with sounds and organizing these letters and sounds to form words. It is a common myth among the public that those with dyslexia see words backwards. Dyslexia is not a visual deficit. When someone with dyslexia writes, letters may be out of order. However, this is related to difficulties with remembering and ordering letters and sounds (language-based) rather than how they may "see" something (visual-based). People with dyslexia may have difficulty with phonological awareness for reading as well as reading decoding and fluency, spelling, and written expression. Oral language deficits are also often present, such as difficulties with retrieval and language organization, which may contribute to difficulties retrieving letter and/or sound names and organizing thoughts for writing (International Dyslexia Association, 2017).

## COMMONLY OCCURRING EXECUTIVE FUNCTIONING DEFICITS IN INDIVIDUALS WITH LEARNING DIFFERENCES

Clients with learning differences can present with difficulties in every area of EF discussed in Chapter 4: self-awareness, self-monitoring, goal setting, attention to task, working memory, phonological encoding, response inhibition, retrieval, cognitive flexibility, problem solving, and task persistence. If a client has a diagnosed learning difference, then they have undergone a full psychological and/or neuropsychological evaluation (which includes intelligence testing), as well as an educational evaluation measuring levels of academic achievement. Reading the reports from these evaluations and/or connecting with the professional conducting them will help educate you as to the areas of EF that are likely to

*There is a parallel between school failure and failure of fluency therapy.*

cause the most difficulty. What tends to happen in the real world is that no client will present with just one of these EF deficits. It is often the combination of several of these areas of deficit that interact and manifest into the client's difficulties with learning. It is important to keep in mind that several may interact and create a response in your client that may vary from one situation to the next. The most helpful

thing the clinician can do is to 1) be aware of the possible EF deficits your client may present with; 2) be watchful for when these deficits occur and/or interact; and 3) be observant about the impact these deficits have upon your client's response to therapy activities. As will be illustrated in the case examples later, the clinician will need to be observant and flexible to identify what is truly going on vs. what might appear on the surface to be something else. The EF deficits that are described will be highlighted as they arise to show the clinician how difficulties in these areas may interfere with progress in therapy.

## EXECUTIVE FUNCTIONING DEFICITS: IDENTIFYING AND DEALING WITH THEM FOR FLUENCY TREATMENT

Some real case examples will illustrate the interaction of different EF deficits and ideas of managing these so that fluency therapy can be as productive as possible. In our university clinic, we had an eighth grader who had been attending literacy sessions for about 2 years. This client had a long-standing history of school failure and was reading at a first-grade level. He had difficulty with letter-sound association, phonological encoding, retrieval, and working memory, which made the task of sounding out words quite laborious for him. He was sent out of his school district to a private school for students with learning differences. Though it was expected he would thrive in this environment, he did not. Rather, teachers said that he lacked motivation to benefit from the instruction he was being given. Eventually he went back to school in his district, where he continued to be labeled as "unmotivated." His mother decided to place him in a private school so that he could have small-group instruction. It was about this time that he came to our university clinic for services. For three semesters, the client's progress was a constant uphill battle. He argued why activities we presented wouldn't work before he even tried them (cognitive flexibility, task persistence, goal setting), while at the same time acknowledging that he would like help to read better. His self-awareness of his difficulties in general was adequate, and he was quite vocal about being baffled when his teachers asked him if because of his dyslexia he "sees things backwards." He was often off task (attention to task) and needed frequent redirection to inhibit responses (response inhibition) about why he didn't enjoy certain activities. Empowering him with activity choices, high-interest content, and discussing all goals and rationales with him did help, but not completely. The fourth semester, the client began to attend group sessions in addition to his individual sessions. He was grouped with another young man of similar age who also had severe reading decoding deficits. Being paired with another student who also experienced the difficulties he did made a huge impact upon this boy's motivation. Without directly discussing it, the client was able to see that others his age also struggled like he did. We went from him arguing about activities to him requesting specific goals for himself (goal setting), such as a spelling goal. The support he gained from the group setting shut down any complaints. Although this was not a fluency client, this is important for the clinician to keep in mind when planning sessions with "resistant" clients who may have experienced either school or therapy failure in the past. It is not uncommon for fluency clients to feel that they are the only ones in their school who are dealing with a fluency disorder. Many reach adulthood and still haven't met someone who stutters or clutters. The case I described illustrates that when schedules and group dynamics allow you to group clients with fluency disorders together, this may be beneficial not just from a planning but also from a motivational perspective. If schedules do not allow for this, making sure that clients with fluency disorders can meet and/or connect (via Internet or in-person support groups, etc.) with others their age who have fluency disorders is extremely important to building and maintaining motivation.

Another case example of a client who initially seemed extremely unmotivated was a client with a language-based learning disorder. The client had difficulties with processing auditory information and retrieving and organizing language output (phonological encoding), ADHD (attention), cluttering and word-final disfluencies. As I have seen this client over a 7-year period for different reasons, it provides a nice illustration of how someone with fluency and concomitant disorders may move through the process of managing their fluency disorders. This young man began therapy with me at age 8. The main focus was upon cluttering and word-final disfluencies, as he was receiving therapy for his other language-based issues at school. I was brought in as the fluency specialist on the case. When I initially began with this client, he did not recognize his role in clear communication (self-awareness, goal setting). If others could not understand him due to cluttering, he often felt that his listener had difficulty hearing, would become frustrated (task persistence), raise his voice, and repeat his sentence at a higher volume (cognitive flexibility, problem solving). Sometimes this higher volume increased clarity; other times it did not. Self-regulation (self-monitoring) was very difficult, and he required frequent redirection and reminders for focus (attention to task). Over time he gradually began to acknowledge that 1) if others didn't understand his message, it likely could be because he was using unclear or "mushy" speech and 2) if he wanted others to understand his message, he needed to not just repeat what he had just said, but repeat it in a different way that would increase understanding (such as emphasizing sounds and syllables, adding in natural pauses to slow rate, etc.). Over time, the client also required more support from me for his difficulties with auditory processing related to classroom activities, such as note taking. By this time, fluency strategies had been learned and just needed to be applied to moments of real communication breakdowns. Therefore, the main focus shifted away from fluency to work on auditory processing strategies, and use of strategies for cluttering and word-final disfluencies was reinforced in the background of other activities. The client attended middle school in a special school that was structured to address his learning needs. His parents honored his wish to transition to a mainstream high school with academic support. He had built a lot of foundation skills at his middle school, and his family hoped he was ready for the change. I continued to reinforce (in the background) use of strategies to repair the communication breakdowns that occur during sessions. However, currently, more of my focus has been upon helping him to manage EF skills due to the increased demands for long-term assignments, studying, and tests/quizzes in his high school. The client is highly motivated and wants to demonstrate to his parents (who worry that mainstream high school may be too overwhelming for him) that he can effectively manage high school. Managing high school includes communicating clearly with others. During a summer program the client attended at his high school before his ninth-grade year, his motivation began to soar. However, two months into the school year, his grades were slipping. He was falling behind on assignments. He was not telling his mother of the daily problems he was having, such as losing his daily planner. When asked about his grades, he said he was having a hard time getting motivated to study (task persistence). His mother remarked that he has always lacked motivation. How does the client, who clearly wants to do well in his new high school, appear so unmotivated? He contends that he still wants to do well in school to show his parents that he can. Is he motivated or just paying lip service to the idea of motivation? In delving a little deeper, I found out that the client felt very overwhelmed with what he hadn't accomplished. He was afraid his parents would be disappointed in him, so he was not telling them of the problems he has (problem solving). He hadn't spoken to his teachers about getting help for two reasons: 1) he was afraid this signaled lack of independence and 2) he was afraid they would not understand his speech. So is he truly unmotivated? No. His difficulties with cognitive flexibility, prioritizing (goal setting), and problem solving were now shining through to illustrate the negative impact these EF deficits can have on client progress. The client needed support from a counselor to help with acceptance of what he needs to do to succeed (self-awareness), as he didn't want to use strategies because he thought that this would illustrate he wasn't independent. He needed help with problem solving to see that by using strategies, he is actually helping to show that he is becoming an independent learner. The point of this illustration is that EF deficits can stall your clients in their progress. To anyone looking from the outside in, the client may truly appear unmotivated. Perhaps they are unmotivated. But to know for sure, we have to figure out why they are unmotivated and help support the client in the appropriate areas. It was not my role as clinician to do the job of the counselor. However, because I subscribe to the philosophy that this client's behavior is telling us something, I spent a lot of time reflecting on why this client might appear unmotivated. I also spent a lot of time asking him closed-ended questions (to support difficulties with retrieval and phonological encoding) to get to the bottom of how he was feeling. It was important for me to keep in mind that when others asked him about his difficulties, he often had problems articulating what these were due to problems with language organization. Because he felt he should answer any questions presented to him, if he could not articulate it accurately, he would choose a simpler response to articulate, even if it wasn't quite accurate (e.g., "I'm not very motivated"). By spending this time talking with the client, I was able to identify the root of the problem, put key professionals and solutions into place, and use the difficulties that arose to increase motivation for fluency work. That is, recall that this client was afraid to communicate with teachers for fear they would not understand his speech. I used the client's concern as a teachable moment to help him learn that using cluttering strategies would assist with teachers understanding him clearly the first time.

A final story in motivation illustrates how strategies presented may not work at a given time even when presented effectively. Sometimes these strategies need to be placed on the back burner until the right moment presents itself. I was working with a 9-year-old boy with word-final disfluencies and a concomitant diagnosis of autism spectrum disorder, level 1. Although he could tell elaborate stories on topics of his own choosing, he often had difficulty separating out the main points from details, and therefore his stories would be bogged down in details that would lose his listener (word retrieval, self-awareness, self-monitoring). Because he presented with increased word-final disfluencies (WFDs) during this storytelling context, I hypothesized that helping him to better organize his thoughts for storytelling would decrease the WFDs. We worked on the idea of pausing to give himself more think time, and he took to this strategy well. One day I presented the concept of visual organizers to plan his story before speaking. He was resistant. He said, "I don't like to plan out my stories, I just like to tell them as they come out" (self-awareness, goal setting, cognitive flexibility). I tried again on other days at other times and received a similar response. I decided that even though I thought this strategy would be quite helpful to my client, forcing him to use it when he didn't buy into it wouldn't serve him well in the long term. One of my philosophies under which I operate with clients is that it's always about how much benefit they can see to using a strategy that results in them putting in the work needed to practice the strategy. He saw no benefit, and likely if I pursued it, wouldn't apply it without cueing from others, and likely that would also bring about resistance. Does this client have difficulty with cognitive flexibility in that he won't even try a new strategy? Absolutely. I decided that I needed to work within his difficulties with flexibility and figure out another way for him to use organizational strategies before speaking. I began to work on visualizing while speaking, which he was slightly more receptive to. In the meantime, we started to play a game where the speaker has to speak on a topic for at least 1 and no more than 2 minutes (see end of chapter). When attempting to decide what to say about a given topic, this client became very frustrated. Any of the topics he typically spoke about with ease, he said he couldn't remember what to say about them (retrieval). This was surprising, but I kept observing the client's reactions. It seemed that when he talked about a topic or told a story on his terms, there was little difficulty in him starting and continuing through to the end. But when he was put on the spot with the same topics, he couldn't come up with what to say (retrieval). I realized he really was stuck. I didn't want to use the word visual organizer, but I thought about how this was the perfect teachable moment to show him the benefits of one. I told him I would ask him questions about a topic and write down notes about his answers so he could use them when it was his turn to tell the story. I asked him concrete questions, he responded, and I wrote down notes on a visual organizer (which was not labeled as such). He used the organizer during his turn with ease. We talked about how it made things easier. The following week when we were ready to play the game again, I reminded him how well he had done the previous week. He asked, "Would you help me write the stuff down again?" Of course I would! This example illustrates how the clinician always needs to be ready to go in one of these moments. It illustrates how the client saw the benefit of the organizer and was motivated to use it again in a real-life situation. It also illustrates how problems in one area of EF can present an opportunity for growth in other areas of EF. When motivation appears lacking, think about what may be underlying the lack of motivation. Is it something that needs to be addressed by other professionals? Is it something that we need to change our plan and see if that helps? By understanding all the EF components that go in to learning, we can better work with and around (if needed) the trouble spots to help our clients get the most benefit from fluency strategies.

# MANAGEMENT STRATEGIES

# LANGUAGE-BASED ACTIVITIES WITH FLUENCY FOCUS (CLUTTERING, STUTTERING, ATYPICAL DISFLUENCIES)

# ACTIVITY 7-1: RETRIEVAL ACTIVITIES WITH FLUENCY FOCUS (CLUTTERING, STUTTERING, ATYPICAL DISFLUENCIES)

Choose one of the activities to work on. All activities help to build word retrieval and language organization. Following the activity are ways to incorporate fluency goals.

- Name items in a given category.
- List three to four subcategories for a given category. (Example: subcategories for "food" might be "breakfast foods," "desserts," "fruits," and "vegetables.")
- List synonyms for given words
- List antonyms for given words.
- Use visual organizers to retell a story. Story elements could include setting, characters, problem, solution, initiating event, or whatever elements were covered in your client's classroom.
- Play a game where the speaker talks about a topic for at least 1 minute (for those who have trouble expanding on thoughts) and no more than 3 minutes (for those who have trouble wrapping thoughts up). Assign fluency goals to use when in the speaker role. When in the listener role, the client can record the number of times the clinician (or other students in the group) use assigned strategies. You can give bonus points for staying within the time and each time a strategy is followed.

*For stuttering*: Client should use preparatory set as they initiate voicing to say each word or as they initiate the start of each phrase or sentence.

*For cluttering*: Client should emphasize endings of each word they say in a natural way, especially multisyllabic words.

*For atypical disfluency*: Client should put natural pauses between each word or phrase they say.

# ACTIVITY 7-2:
# ACTIVITIES FOR AUDITORY PROCESSING WITH FLUENCY FOCUS (CLUTTERING, STUTTERING, ATYPICAL DISFLUENCIES)

What follows are activities which combine fluency strategies with language-based activities. Before your client can work on auditory processing disorders, they need to be educated about what they are dealing with at a level they can understand. Remember that students with learning disabilities have average to above-average IQ scores. Therefore, any client with diagnosed learning disabilities should be able to follow the information presented here. Clinicians can make the information more concrete if they feel this is needed, especially for clients of younger ages. I find this activity to be most appropriate starting at age 8 or 9.

For the activity "What Is Auditory Processing?" you can have your client reiterate what is explained in the handout as if conveying the information to a teacher or other professional. I often like to have my students with learning disabilities role-play how they might explain their difficulties to a teacher who has little experience with this disorder. Practicing in a safe environment helps clients start to get used to advocating for themselves, a skill that they will need to master and use throughout their academic career. When presented in simple terms, I find students can start to role-play at age 8 or 9. This is a good context to practice fluency strategies in connected speech. For example, they can use preparatory set at the start of each phrase or sentence, use natural pausing throughout their explanation, and/or emphasize ending sounds. They can practice looking for feedback from the listener to make sure that their speech is clear and that their listener is following them.

## What Is Auditory Processing?

Auditory processing is how your brain understands what you hear.

If you have trouble with auditory processing, it is not because you are not as smart as other people.

If you have trouble with auditory processing, it just means that your brain sometimes has trouble understanding directions exactly. This might be because the directions are too long or too complicated.

**Student Activity**: Complete the following statements, and act out explaining this to your teacher, who will play the role of different teachers. Remember that some teachers may have a harder time than others understanding what auditory processing is. You and your speech teacher can practice explaining these things to teachers who will understand quickly and others who will need more explanation.

These are the things that are more difficult for me in school because of my auditory processing disorder:

These are the things that help me the most when I am having a hard time processing:

# ACTIVITY 7-3:
# KEY WORDS AND NOTE TAKING FOR AUDITORY PROCESSING

Whenever a clinician is working on auditory processing, they want to think about the contexts in which a client may need to process information for school or work settings. In both settings, there may be times when the client needs to take notes. Many clients with auditory processing disorders struggle with selecting the key information. Therefore, introducing the client to key words is important. Use the following activity to introduce what key words are. Have the client practice highlighting or circling key words in written sentences. Once the client demonstrates comprehension of this concept, present the sentences auditorily and have them repeat key words back to you using fluency strategies.

## What Are Key Words?

Key words are the words that carry meaning in a sentence. If you take key words out of a sentence, you will lose the original meaning. Often key words represent nouns and verbs.

**Example**: Go to the store and buy some bread.
**Key words**: go store buy bread

Whether I say, "Go to the store and buy some bread" or "Go store buy bread," the listener gets the same meaning. Although key words are not the way we would write an essay, they are helpful to focus on when listening to directions. If we focus on the key words, it is less work for our listening brains, and we get the main message more easily. The less important words in a sentence are often articles and connector words, such as "and" and "the." However, be careful to make sure that if you remove one of these words, the meaning doesn't change. For example:

You will get a toy if you are good.
You get toy good.

If we remove "if" from this sentence, a key piece of meaning is lost. Does "You get toy good" mean you will get a good toy? It's good you'll get a toy? Something else? What the client should remember is that there is no hard-and-fast rule for the types of words that are most important. This really does depend on the sentence. The client can test this out by reading the original sentence, then the key word sentence, and making sure no meaning is lost. They can do this using fluency strategies as well!

# ACTIVITY 7-4:
# SELF-REGULATION

Following is an activity you can use to have your client work on self-regulation. Once the concepts are presented, the client can reiterate the learned concepts using fluency strategies. The clinician can also have the client answer questions about the concepts using fluency strategies during a structured game.

For more practice using fluency strategies in longer utterances, the clinician can:

- Provide problem situations related to the following concepts and have the client explain solutions and their rationales using fluency strategies.

- Seize upon teachable moments where the client did not follow these rules and misunderstood the information. The clinician could have the client explain what went wrong and what could be done better next time while using fluency strategies.

These are the things I need to do in order to process information I hear correctly:

- **Ignore** distractions

  ○ In my mind

  ○ Around me (things I can see, smell, or hear)

- **Control** my impulses

  ○ Think, "Is this a good idea?" BEFORE I act or speak.

  ○ If it is NOT a good idea, then do NOT say it or do it.

- **Process** the information

  ○ If I don't understand, I should ask for help processing the information.

# ACTIVITY 7-5:
# ACTIVE AND PASSIVE LEARNERS

## What Does It Mean to Be a Passive Learner?

This means that when you don't understand something, you don't do anything about it. You don't understand, but you don't ask questions. You just do whatever you think should be done, even if you're not sure if it's right.

Sometimes when the teacher is just talking and not asking you a question, you could become a passive learner. You could just let your mind go blank and then you won't process what the teacher is saying. Even though the teacher is not asking you a question, there are negative consequences if you don't process the information. You might not understand the directions, or you might miss out on learning something very important.

It is normal for everyone's mind to go blank sometimes when listening. This is not something people do on purpose, but it does happen and they miss information. When someone realizes that their mind has gone blank, they need to tell the person and politely ask them to repeat the information.

## What Does It Mean to Be an Active Learner?

The way to prevent your mind from going blank as much as possible is to do active listening. This means that you are focusing on what the other person is saying and really thinking about what they say. If you are confused about what they are saying, you take initiative and ask them about it. You keep your mind active so your brain is really thinking about and processing the information.

## Why Should I Care About This Anyway?

Kids who have trouble with auditory processing have to work extra hard to process information. Their brains get tired. So their brains like to try and take breaks and go passive while listening. But this is not a good idea! By working hard at active listening, you can take control and help your brain process the information. If you process it the first time, you will have less work to do to try and understand the information later.

Answer the following questions by talking them out with your speech clinician. Use your fluency strategies while you are talking.

**My plan for active listening:**


List three topics where your brain likes to try and take a break and go blank.
1.

2.

3.


List three classes or activities at school where your brain likes to try and take a break and go blank.
1.

2.

3.

List three topics where your brain never seems to go blank.

1.

2.

3.

List three activities at school where your brain never seems to go blank.

1.

2.

3.

Answer the following questions by talking them out with your speech clinician. Use your fluency strategies while you are talking.

**My active learning and passive learning for the week of:**

List three times this week when your mind went blank and you did nothing (passive learner).

1.

2.

3.

List three times this week when your mind went blank and what you did about it (active learner).

1.

2.

3.

Name a topic that was easy for you to focus on without your mind going blank:

Rate how much effort you had to put in to keep focused on the topic
(1= very little effort; 10 = a lot of effort):

Name a topic that was difficult for you to focus on without your mind going blank:

Rate how much effort you had to put in to keep focused on the topic
(1= very little effort; 10 = a lot of effort):

# ACTIVITY 7-6:
# IDENTIFYING AND PROBLEM SOLVING DIFFICULTIES IN AUDITORY PROCESSING

When clients have difficulty with processing auditory information, the first step is for them to identify when a breakdown in processing occurs so that they can repair the breakdown as needed. Clients may start this process by identifying and saying something general such as, "I didn't get that." This is a great first step in repairing the communication breakdown. Ultimately, the client needs to give more specific information to the speaker about what they missed so that the most efficient repair can be made (e.g., repeating the last piece of information said rather than the entire thing). Figure 7-1 shows a flow chart I use to help the client identify potential specific sources of breakdown in processing. To incorporate fluency strategies, the client can explain things on the flow chart after concepts have been presented, teaching others about what they have learned. Or the clinician and client can watch instances of processing breakdowns on video and identify what the listener should have done (or did do if applicable) to repair the breakdown. Ultimately, as processing breakdowns occur in the course of other activities, the client can use the flow chart to identify what happened and a potential solution. All discussions, role plays, and applications to real life can involve reinforcement of fluency strategies.

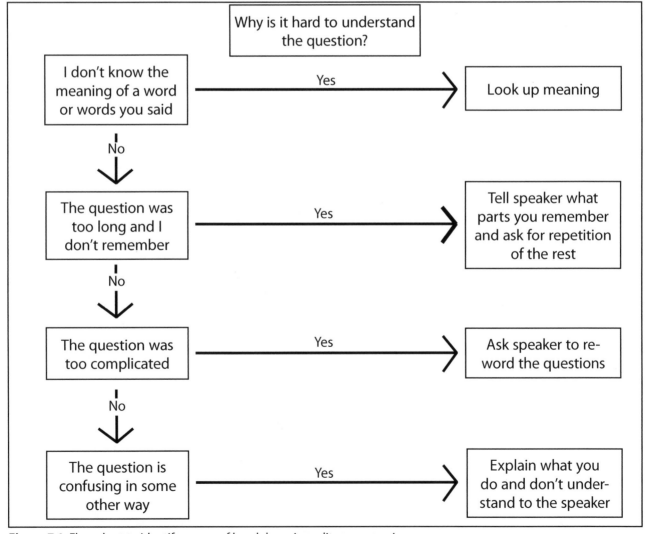

**Figure 7-1.** Flow chart to identify source of breakdown in auditory processing.

As with the earlier activities, after the following concepts have been presented and understood, the client can incorporate fluency strategies into the following activities:

- Discussing the concepts presented

- Teaching or explaining the concepts to someone else

- Answering questions about the concepts during a game

- Verbalizing how to apply the concepts to real situations

# ACTIVITY 7-7:
# WHAT IS LANGUAGE ORGANIZATION?

Language organization is how well language is organized in your mind. When information is well organized, you can find it easily. When information is not well organized, you have trouble finding it quickly. This can make these things difficult:

- Thinking of a word you want to say

- Organizing a lot of information, like you would have to do when explaining something complicated

- Organizing a lot of information, like you would have to do when writing

## *Why Do Some Kids Have Trouble With Language Organization?*

The words are just not well organized in their minds. It is not their fault; it just happens this way.

## *What Can Help With Language Organization?*

If you can't think of a word, describing the word you are trying to think of helps.

If you have a hard time explaining something, having an outline in your head helps.

If you have a hard time thinking of what to write about, using some kind of outline or story map helps.

If you have a hard time expanding on your ideas, what can help?

- Answer who, what, where, when, why, and how questions.

- Talk about all five senses. Tell what you hear, see, touch, taste, and smell.

# MELDING LITERACY AND FLUENCY WORK TOGETHER

The remainder of this chapter deals with phonological awareness, reading decoding, reading fluency, and reading comprehension strategies. They are provided for those clinicians who may do less work with learning disabilities, and need some ideas about melding fluency and literacy goals together. Depending on your work setting, you may not need to address the reading goals, but using the context of reading with a client who is struggling in this area may be beneficial. Just be sure that before you start incorporating fluency concepts into these very difficult aspects of reading, the fluency concepts have been mastered. In this way, the client can practice fluency strategies during any of the activities at just the right challenge. Please note that the information below was written so that it can be easily used with beginning clinicians you may be supervising.

## *Things I Need to Know About Evaluating and Working With Phonological Awareness*

### What Is Phonological Awareness?

Phonological awareness (PA) is a child's ability to be aware of the sounds letters make and their ability to manipulate letters and sounds/syllables in words. These skills should be fully developed by age 10 (although most are developed much earlier) and form the foundations of being able to manipulate letters and sounds for reading and spelling. Examples of phonological awareness skills are the ability to identify whether or not two words rhyme; make up a new rhyming word from a given word; identify beginning, middle, and ending sounds in words; blend phonemes together to make words; name the sounds that each letter makes; and manipulate syllables/sounds to make new words.

Some children may not have really strong PA skills but are strong readers. These children tend to be known as "whole word readers" and do not need PA therapy. However, many children with PA issues are at risk for later reading and spelling difficulties. Some kids with poor PA who are strong readers may need more help with reading decoding and/or spelling as they move into fourth grade and beyond, when they can no longer rely on just sight to read and spell more complicated words.

### How Can I Tell If My Client Has Trouble With Phonological Awareness?

If they had an evaluation already, look to see if the Phonological Awareness Test, Second Edition (PAT-2) or a similar test of phonological awareness was part of the tests administered.

If it was, look to see the sections where your client had trouble. On the PAT-2, the skills are grouped in sections by approximate developmental order. Whatever sections your client has trouble with (i.e., gets three or more wrong), that is the target skill you will address in therapy. So, for example, if your client got 7/10 correct on naming rhyming words, you might write the following short-term goal:

*When presented with an age-appropriate word by the clinician, the client will name an appropriate rhyming word with 90% accuracy and minimal clinician cues.*

Think about what skill the sections of the PAT-2 your client has trouble with is targeting. For example, if your client had trouble with phoneme deletion (say "pat," now say it without the /p/) and phoneme substitution (say "fall," now change the /f/ to /b/), these are both forms of phoneme manipulation. So you might write the following short-term goal:

*Client will complete phoneme manipulation activities (including phoneme deletion and phoneme substitution) with 90% accuracy and minimal clinician cueing.*

Remember that you can use the concepts of the items presented on the PAT-2, but don't just use the examples the child got wrong on the test in therapy. Make up your own new examples for therapy sessions.

Be specific in your goal writing, so that only the skills your client has trouble with are targeted. Remember that kids with learning differences tend to have "holes" you need to fill. So if your client had trouble naming the sound that went with diphthongs and digraphs in isolation but not in naming long and short vowels or consonants, then you only target where they had trouble. In that case, your short-term goal might say:

*Client will name sound when presented with specific letter combinations (digraphs, diphthongs) with 90% accuracy and minimal clinician cues.*

Remember to put the specific patterns that should be targeted in therapy in your goal!

If your client has not been evaluated with the PAT-2 and you want to know if your client (between ages 5 and 9 years) has trouble with phonological awareness, administer the PAT-2. Any section your client got three or more wrong on you will target for a goal, as explained earlier.

Note for older students: Similar skills are targeted on the Comprehensive Test of Phonological Processing, Second Edition (CTOPP-2) for children older than age 9. Look at the PA skills the PAT-2 targets and find similar subtests on the CTOPP-2. If after testing you find your client has trouble with phonological awareness, goals can be targeted as described earlier.

## Things I Need to Know About Word Study

### What Is Word Study?

Word study is a way for students to analyze words and figure out patterns of reading and spelling rules. The idea of word study is for a student to start to see patterns in words so that they can start using strategies to decode and encode (spell) words on their own more efficiently. Instead of trying to sound out each sound individually, they start to see larger patterns in words and can decode them more quickly and accurately.

### How Do I Write a Short-Term Goal for Word Study?

See what reading rules they had trouble with on the last two sections of the PAT-2 and/or the Gray Oral Reading Test, Fifth Edition (GORT-5), or a similar test that looks at reading decoding skills. Use those rules for your word study activity. Examples of rules:

- Silent e at the end of a word makes the vowel say its name:

  **Example**: "cave"; e makes "a" say its name and become long "a"
- Two vowels go walking, the first one does the talking:

  **Examples**: "ai" like in "sail"; "ea" like in "eat"
- The letter "c" makes the /s/ sound when followed by i, e, or y (city, cyberspace, ceiling). When followed by any other vowels, it makes the /k/ sound (cat, cot, cut).
- The letter "g" makes the "j" sound when followed by i, e, or y (giant, gem, gym). When followed by any other vowels, it makes the "g" sound (game, gum, gone).
- "er," "ir," and "ur" all make the same sound, "er."
- "oi" and "oy" make the same sound.

Based upon the rules your client has trouble with on testing, you can write a general goal for word study, but include specifics in it so the clinician knows exactly what patterns to target in therapy.

*Client will complete word study activities (focusing on vowel digraphs, silent e) with 90% accuracy with minimal clinician cueing.*

Following is an example of a word study activity focusing on the vowel digraphs:

- Make nine index cards:
  - ◦ Three with words containing ai (rain, main, train)
  - ◦ Three with words that contain ea (read, eat, beat)
  - ◦ Three with words that contain oa (boat, coat, soap)
- Underline the key letters in each word (ai, oa, ea).
- Mix the cards up and tell client she doesn't need to be able to read all the words, but she has to look at the underlined letters and see if she can sort the cards into three different groups.
- Once she has them sorted, talk about the sounds that each pair of letters make. Help her to deduce that in each set of 3 cards, when two vowels are together, the first one says its name. Write out a reading rule for vowel digraphs, wording this as the client's classroom teacher does (e.g., "Two vowels go walking the first one does the talking"). Include the rule in the binder described below.

## Using a Binder

Ask the caregiver if they can bring in a binder with five dividers for the next session. One of the tabs will be "reading rules" (other tabs will be "homework," "completed homework," and "strategies"; leave the fifth one blank). You'll make a handout that reviews what digraphs are in language the client can understand to refer back to.

Spend about 15 minutes on word study each week.

Kids with reading issues need lots of repetition, review, and reinforcement.

- Always review what you worked on the previous week for just a few minutes at the start of each session.

Kids with reading issues also often don't apply rules to the context of real reading.

- Once you have completed a word study activity, see the following section for "Applying Reading Rules in Context."

# APPLYING READING RULES IN CONTEXT

## Why Is This Important?

Because students with reading issues often have trouble applying the rules they learn to the context of real reading.

## What Would a Short-Term Goal Look Like for This?

*Client will apply reading rules to age-appropriate reading activities with 90% accuracy and minimal clinician cues.*

In your other reading decoding goals for the client, you should have specified what those rules the child is working on are. But if you didn't specify, be sure to do so here. Remember, kids with learning differences need you to fill the missing "holes," so it is very important that you identify and know where those holes are.

## What Does an Activity for This Goal Look Like?

It's a good idea to have the reading rules you have gone over in a binder for the client to keep building upon. The binder allows you and the client to refer back to the rules you learned as they apply to real reading. The client will not be able to keep all of these rules in their head, so having a binder of the rules is an invaluable reference. See the section on word study for more information about how to organize the binder.

Bring in a book appropriate for client's age and reading level. If you have time, call the caregiver before the session and have them bring in a book the child likes or is reading for school. For future sessions you can have your client always bring a book from home or school. In this way, you can reinforce what your client is really reading.

If the book is at your client's reading level, you can take turns reading a page of the book. When one person is reading, the listener is looking for examples of words containing sounds you focused on in your word study during the session. So if you focused on "ai" words, your client tries to find all the words that contain "ai" on the page you are reading. Keep in mind your client's comprehension of the page may not be too strong because they are focused on finding word patterns. That is fine because your focus is on applying reading decoding rules to real reading. Your focus here is not on comprehension, so don't worry about that for this activity. As your client finds the words, they write them on paper. Then after you read the page, you talk about the words they found and what sounds they make (e.g., "Oh, you found 'eat'; the 'e' says its name").

Keep in mind that your client may have trouble finding words as you read at first. If they do, you can prompt them by saying, for example, "I see a word on this line." Point out the line it is on and see if that helps them find it. If they still have trouble, say, "It's between these two words," etc. Obviously if there are no words on the page fitting the pattern you are looking for, you move on to reading the next page.

If your client is using a book they can easily decode, you can write down words while they read a page. If they like competition, you can "compete" to see who can find more words while the other person reads. Or you can see how many words you can both find together and add them to a big list (e.g., "Our 'ai' words") sorted into categories by sounds they make. In future weeks, see if you can make longer lists and break your group record.

## What Is Reading Comprehension?

Reading comprehension is the ability to understand what you read. There are two kinds of reading comprehension:
1. Understanding the literal facts about what you read (e.g., character names, ages, places characters go, dates, etc.).
2. Higher-level comprehension skills. These skills require a reader to take the basic facts of a story as well as any word and/or picture clues to:
   ◦ Make predictions about what will happen next
   ◦ Draw conclusions/make inferences about how a character is feeling
   ◦ Identify the main idea of a nonfiction piece or the main events of a short story or chapter of a longer story

## What Are Some Reasons a Student Might Have Trouble With Reading Comprehension?

The main failure in comprehension of literal facts is the ability to picture something as you read it. There are several underlying reasons a student might have trouble with picturing sentences as they read them. Remember that a student may have more than one contributing factor to this difficulty. Examples of reasons why a client might have difficulty picturing what they read include the following:

- They do not understand the meaning of vocabulary in the passage they are reading. You can't picture a word you don't understand and/or have never heard before. Or, the client might confuse the meaning of one word with another (e.g., "plains" vs. "planes"), picture the wrong meaning of the word, and thereby inaccurately picture the story.
- They do not have enough background information on the topic (e.g., a student who has never seen what an irrigation system looks like would have a very hard time picturing this even if the word "irrigation" was defined for them).
- They have difficulties with memory for details. You can't picture what you can't remember.
- They have difficulty understanding complex syntax. For example, if you think that the sentence written in passive voice "The boy was helped by the girl" means that the boy helped the "girl," then you are going to misunderstand the meaning of what happened.

If you have trouble with remembering and/or comprehending the facts of the story, you will be unable to use these facts for higher-level reading comprehension, such as making predictions, drawing conclusions, and stating the main idea. You need to be able to put the basic facts together from a story to draw conclusions, make predictions, etc. Once a client has understanding and recall of the basic facts of the story, reasons they might still have trouble with higher-level reading comprehension skills include the following:

- They have overall difficulty focusing on relevant information when they read. That is to say that they get bogged down in details and give all details of what they read "equal weight" or importance. This often results in difficulties with identifying the main idea or title of a story.
- They do not understand how to use the actual words (e.g., excited, sad, frustrated), picture clues, and/or text and punctuation (e.g., exclamation points, all caps, or bold print) to help them "read between the lines" of the facts and draw a conclusion. They often miss these clues and need them to be explicitly taught to use them.

## How Can I Tell If My Client Has Trouble With Reading Comprehension?

If they had an evaluation already, look to see if the GORT-5 or another test of reading comprehension was part of the tests administered.

If it was, look for patterns in the types of comprehension questions your client got wrong. The GORT-5 asks two types of reading comprehension questions: factual and higher-level comprehension (both described earlier). Whatever sections your client has trouble with (i.e., has a pattern of getting most of the factual questions right but most of the higher-level comprehension questions wrong), that is the target skill you will address in therapy. So, for example, if your client was having trouble with recall of factual information, you might write the following short-term goal:

*When presented with an age-appropriate short story by the clinician, the client will answer factual comprehension questions with 90% accuracy and minimal clinician cues.*

If your client was having trouble with higher-level comprehension questions, think about what specific reading comprehension skills the sections of the GORT-5 your client had trouble with are targeting. For example, if your client had trouble with identifying the main idea and inferring questions, you would write the following short-term goal:

*When presented with an age-appropriate short story by the clinician, the client will answer higher-level comprehension questions (i.e., identifying main idea, making inferences) with 90% accuracy and minimal clinician cues.*

If your client has not been evaluated with the GORT-5 or some other test of reading comprehension and you want to know if your client has trouble with reading comprehension, administer a test that measures this. You will write goals based upon the patterns of errors you see in their comprehension questions, as explained earlier.

**Note**: While you are administering the GORT-5, you will want to gain qualitative information to help you determine the root of why your client cannot answer questions accurately. Observe the client as they approach the question and look for patterns. For example, do they often ask you to define a word in the question? Although you cannot define the word when administering the test in the standardized way, this pattern tells you that vocabulary issues might be relating to difficulties with reading comprehension. Another thing you might notice is that the child asks you if they can go back and look for the answer in the story. Although you cannot allow them to do this when administering the test the standardized way, this pattern tells you that memory issues might be relating to difficulties with reading comprehension.

Note that after you have given the test the standardized way, you can go back to questions the client missed and see if scaffolding certain areas you suspect as areas of difficulty help them to answer correctly. For example, if you allow them to look back at the text for an answer to a comprehension question and this often seems to help them, you might suspect an issue with auditory memory. If you define a word they don't understand and this helps them to answer the question correctly, you might suspect an issue with vocabulary. If you reword a complex question for them and this helps them to answer the question correctly, you might suspect they have difficulty with processing/understanding complex syntax. The Qualitative Reading Inventory is a standardized test that also measures many of these skills.

## Methods for Treating Reading Comprehension Issues

Once you have identified the reading comprehension issues, you need to work on what you have identified as the key issues. If you just start having a client read and answer questions in therapy, without understanding why they cannot answer the questions, then you are not really working on the root cause of their reading comprehension issues, and you likely will see little carryover of skills. You need to target your therapy according to where the breakdown in skills is. So if your student has trouble with picturing the basic facts of the story, try to figure out why. Treat and adapt your activity according to the reasons for the breakdown.

For example, if they seem to have trouble understanding vocabulary and/or background information, go through the story you will present them with beforehand and pre-teach difficult vocabulary words/new concepts. By pre-teaching, don't just give them written/verbal definitions of words or concepts. You need to show them pictures of new vocabulary words and concepts and relate the vocabulary/concepts to their life experience to help them really understand the meaning prior to reading the passage. For older students, you will teach them how to go through a story before reading and scan for words/concepts they may need more background information on.

If they seem to have trouble recalling details of the story/passage read, you can work with your client on filling in a story map while reading and referring to this after reading.

If they seem to have difficulties with complex syntax in passages and/or questions, you need to work on understanding complex syntax. Figure out what specific things they have trouble with (passive voice? complex sentences?) and work specifically on those skills. You can use real reading text to make this more functional, but you will have to choose text that targets their particular area of difficulty.

If your client has trouble with higher-level thinking questions, you will need to work specifically on skills like predicting, inferring, and drawing conclusions.

# CHAPTER 8

# ATTENTION DEFICIT HYPERACTIVITY DISORDER

## DEFINITIONS

Attention deficit hyperactivity disorder (ADHD) is defined as a pattern of inattention and/or impulsivity that significantly interferes with daily functioning. Depending on the criteria met, a person may be diagnosed with a "predominantly inattentive presentation," a "predominantly hyperactive/impulsive presentation," or a "combined presentation" (American Psychiatric Association, 2013). Symptoms may present as mild, moderate, or severe. Additionally, there are some who are diagnosed with a more non-specific attention disorder when they do not meet all criteria for ADHD but have significant impact upon daily functioning (American Psychiatric Association, 2013).

## WHAT FLUENCY ISSUES ARE COMMONLY FOUND IN THIS POPULATION?

As mentioned, there is co-occurrence between fluency disorders and attention disorders (Arndt & Healey, 2001; Blood, Blood, & Tellis, 1999; Blood, Ridenour, Qualls, & Hammer, 2003). Additionally, our initial research work testing the skills of those with atypical disfluency show difficulties with working memory, a known area of deficit in ADHD (Sutkowski, Tokach, & Scaler Scott, 2015). Although attention was not measured specifically by our testing, qualitatively, many in our sample required redirection to task. Parents of the majority of our sample reported difficulties with filtering internal distractions. As will be discussed later in this chapter, these difficulties with inhibiting responses such as responses to internal distractions are proposed to be a key area of deficit in ADHD (Barkley, 2005). Be it a formal diagnosis of ADHD or more subtle observations of attentional weaknesses, a clinician can expect to potentially work with a fluency client who also has difficulties with attention.

Scaler Scott, K.
*Fluency Plus: Managing Fluency Disorders in*
*Individuals With Multiple Diagnoses (pp 131-142).*
© 2018 Taylor & Francis Group.

# MYTHS AND FACTS REGARDING FLUENCY TREATMENT IN ATTENTION DISORDERS

One myth about the ADHD population is that all clients with this difficulty will be either 1) frequently up and out of their seat and impulsive or 2) quietly inattentive. Although clients can exhibit one or the other of these characteristics, they can also exhibit both types. The current diagnostic criteria for ADHD under the fifth edition of the *Diagnostic and Statistical Manual of Mental Disorders* (American Psychiatric Association, 2013) divides ADHD into three subcategories: 1) predominantly inattentive (ADHD-I), 2) predominantly hyperactive/impulsive (ADHD-HI), and 3) combined type (ADHD-C). The third type meets the diagnostic criteria for both types I and II. It is important to keep in mind that clients who are inattentive can also be quietly impulsive. This impulsivity may lead to them to becoming quietly distracted. For example, one student with more outward impulse control issues might blurt out an irrelevant response during a conversation. The impulse was there for the client to make the comment, and they were unable to inhibit that impulse. In the same way, a client may have difficulty inhibiting the impulse to think about something else during a conversation. In both cases, impulse control is a problem and results in inattention to the relevant topic. But because of the outward disruption of the first case, it may be thought that only the first student has difficulties with impulse control.

It is important to keep in mind that clients with ADHD are not lazy, though their inconsistent performance often makes others question whether they are, because it is difficult to understand how the client can use strategies some of the time and not others. Remember that behavioral responses do not occur in a vacuum, and there is so much about differences in situations that may change a client's response from one situation to another. Think about a time when someone has done something that has annoyed you, but you've known it was best to keep it to yourself, so you do. When thinking about your response, you tell yourself you have great self-regulation skills. But take the same situation and add to it that you have gotten little sleep the night before, have a pounding headache, and have a looming work deadline to complete. You want to refrain from responding to the person who has annoyed you, but you don't. Should we say that your poor self-regulation was just an act and that you can control it when you want to? Are you just lazy? Afterward, you regret your actions, as well-intentioned clients with ADHD often do. This example illustrates how even with the best of intentions, our responses may not be consistent. For someone with ADHD, their system is taxed more than the average person. Although we cannot allow their diagnosis to give them a pass on behaving according to social norms, it can help us better understand where the lapses in appropriate response are coming from.

> *Clients with ADHD are not lazy, though their inconsistent performance often makes others question whether they are.*

It is also important to keep in mind that what makes someone with ADHD different are differences in brain function (Barkley, 2005). It has been proposed that in ADHD, the mind is always seeking stimulation. This is known as the delay aversion hypothesis (see Antrop et al., 2006, for review) and states that because those with ADHD have a hard time with delays, they will seek more frequent short-term rewards over long-term rewards. When studies have added stimulation to the wait time, those with ADHD have been found to increase their ability to wait for long-term rewards. Therefore, a client may want to ignore distractions or wait for directions rather than react impulsively, but their biological makeup doesn't allow them to do so. If they increase their level of effort, they may be able to control these impulses and this distractibility. Some situations may make it easier for them to self-monitor than others.

# EXECUTIVE FUNCTIONING ISSUES IN ATTENTION DEFICIT HYPERACTIVITY DISORDER AND WAYS OF MANAGING THEM

## *Scheduling Therapy*

It is well established that those with ADHD have difficulties with executive functioning. The most common areas of difficulty include inhibiting responses (otherwise known as impulse control or response inhibition); attending to task; and skills related to planning, organizing, and following through on tasks. Because of the difficulties with delay aversion mentioned at the start of this chapter, scheduling those clients with ADHD in smaller groups will ensure they have less wait time between turns in the group. The larger the groups and the longer the wait time, the more your client may be likely to seek off-task stimulation, whether that be daydreaming about a different topic, providing an off-topic response, or fidgeting with other available materials.

*Those with ADHD are also known to have difficulty with allocating effort and task persistence (see Barkley, 2005, for review).*

## *During Treatment*

If a client is in a distracting environment, there may be a great deal their brain wants to attend to. Beyond the basics of reducing stimulation in the environment for someone with ADHD, it is important to realize how the concept of the brain seeking new input and stimulation may affect progress in therapy. Increasing stimulation for the task you are working on and the pace of the session may help. As a clinician, it has always intrigued me when some children get close to meeting a goal and then seem to regress. The client is making steady progress and perhaps only has to achieve 90% accuracy one more time before a goal is met. It is at this point that the client starts performing poorly. A thought about this related to our clients with ADHD is that when they get close to mastery, their brains have tired of the activity or concept and are therefore seeking something new. It may not be that they have "forgotten" the concepts presented, but that their brains have moved on, and therefore they are less invested in their accuracy at this point. To compensate for this, I have found it's best to build in a reward system not just for effort, but also for achieving their goals. Building in reminders (visual, verbal) of how close they are to meeting their goal each week and linking the reward to achieving the goal will help with long-term investment. Those with ADHD are also known to have difficulty with allocating effort and task persistence (see Barkley, 2005, for review). Therefore, they may have allocated all of their effort to the first few presentations of the activity and then "run out of steam." Helping to pace both the content of sessions (moving from easy to more challenging back to easy tasks) and the level of effort may help your clients with ADHD maintain focus on their goals and tasks and persist even when tasks become more difficult. When possible, scheduling clients for shorter blocks of time more frequently throughout the week rather than one longer session may help with task persistence.

### Impulse Control

Impulse control is another issue that may interfere with learning fluency techniques. Here is an example of how an exchange might go between a clinician and a client with impulse control difficulties.

**Clinician**: Today we are going to work on stuttering strategies. We are going to do prep set first. You are going to stretch the first vowel in the word. Let's do an example. Let me do it first. We'll say "dad."

**Client**: d-d-d-dad
**Clinician**: Wait for me to show you. Now we'll say "daa—"
**Client**: dad
**Clinician**: Wait for me to show you. Daaaad.
**Client**: Daaad.
**Clinician**: Good. Now try it again and make sure to—
**Client**: Daad.
**Clinician**: Okay, a little—
**Client**: Daaad.

This example illustrates how the client misses critical instruction and cues for effective strategy practice due to impulsivity. If they wait the first time the strategy is presented, then they learn to produce it once. But if the clinician wishes to give further instruction to tweak the strategy practice (as is typically necessary with any clients), the client misses these nuances and may in fact be practicing errors. In an effort to help with lack of impulse control, I use the concept presented at the end of this chapter entitled,

*Impulse control is another issue that may interfere with learning fluency techniques.*

"Extra Effort Saves Me Time." This teaches the client that often when they jump ahead, trying to predict the directions or cues a clinician is attempting to give, they may end up with an inaccurate prediction, and therefore have to try the exercise again. I stress that this is unnecessary work and that they are not gaining any time. Whereas they feel that if they speed ahead it will move them ahead faster, often speeding ahead only slows them

down, as they often have to backtrack until they execute the directions correctly to fix the incorrect practice. Often I will have them complete a task impulsively on purpose, then go back and correct errors and time how long it takes them. Then I will have them complete the same or similar task very carefully, checking work before saying they are done. The second task is also timed and the times are compared. In most cases we see that the extra effort saves clients time in the long run. This makes the concept more concrete for clients. The clinician could use a written task (like writing a sentence quickly) or a task where you are giving verbal directions and they are attempting to jump in and predict them (be sure not to make your directions too predictable). We talk about ways for caregivers to reinforce this concept at home. For example, when a child takes their time on homework and checks it carefully, they often don't have to go back and correct as many items (if any at all). See the handout for "Extra Effort Saves Me Time" at the end of this chapter.

## Working Memory

Another area of difficulty known to coexist in ADHD is working memory. How this manifests itself in relation to the fluency disorder will vary by client. Some clients with ADHD will have a hard time keeping their train of thought, resulting in multiple revisions. What I have found commonly in clients with ADHD, regardless of the type of disfluency presented, is that they have a hard time remembering to use their strategies in structured practice. For example, you may ask a client to use a given strategy while playing a game or having a conversation with you. The client may have every intention of using the strategy. However, after one or two turns in the game or after about 30 seconds of a conversation, the client may forget to continue to use strategies. This may also occur at home. What can be helpful is establishing a nonverbal signal with the client that you can also have significant others use at home. However, be sure that due to difficulties with working memory, the client doesn't forget what the signal is for a few minutes into the activity. I once had a client who I kept signaling to use his fluency strategy of pullout and he wasn't responding to the signal. I stopped and asked if he had seen the signal. He replied that he had. I asked then why he wasn't responding with his strategy. He replied that he was.

I then asked what strategy he was using, and his reply indicated that although we had talked about it at the outset, after a few minutes into the activity, he had forgotten what the signal was for and was responding to what he now "assumed" the signal was for. This example illustrates how it is so important to constantly check in with clients, and if working memory deficits are known or suspected, to provide as many written reminders of cues as possible.

## Self-Regulation

Another thing to keep in mind with the ADHD population is that they do not always use self-talk (an internal motivator) to regulate and reward their progress as others without ADHD might do (Barkley, 2005). Children without ADHD have been reported to begin to develop internal speech as a behavior regulator at age 3 and continue to build on this ability through age 12. Children with ADHD are reported to have delays in this development of self-talk, but the extent of delays is currently unclear. Barkley (2005) believes self-talk is the foundation for development of working memory. Given their difficulties with work-

> *Another thing to keep in mind with the ADHD population is that they do not always use self-talk (an internal motivator) to regulate and reward their progress as others without ADHD might do (Barkley, 2005).*

ing memory and delayed ability to use self-talk, children with ADHD may not use the same techniques that children without ADHD do to persist through a less-than-interesting task. That is, children without ADHD may subvocally encourage themselves and hold their goal and potential reward in mind, whereas children with ADHD may have a harder time doing this (Barkley, 2005). Losing sight of their goal and reward and failure to use self-talk to keep going may cause your client with ADHD to lose motivation, even if doing well in the session. For the self-talk and reminders of rewards, you can, of course, verbally encourage, as speech-language clinicians are well versed at doing: "You already finished five! Only five more to go! You're working so hard! Just five more and you earn your prize!" But for some clients, having the prize in sight as a visual reminder may be needed to bridge the gap for task persistence. I prefer to build internal motivation than to use external rewards. However, for my clients with ADHD, I have sometimes found that external rewards are more helpful in keeping them focused to task and motivated to keep challenging themselves throughout the session.

It has been proposed that those with ADHD have a poor sense of time. Barkley (2005) proposes that the core deficit in those with ADHD is that of inhibiting behavioral responses. Difficulties in this area are thought to lead to difficulties in four primary areas of executive function: nonverbal working memory, verbal working memory, shifting responses, and self-regulation. The individual with ADHD must inhibit primary responses (Barkley, 2005). For example, if the individual has to complete an uninteresting task, they have to inhibit responses that would foster escape from the task, such as becoming distracted by a more desirable activity. Perhaps the individual doesn't inhibit the desire to escape and becomes wrapped up in a more

> *Keeping a "just right" pace in terms of interest and your client's ability to process, using visuals to remind your client of their short-term goals within the session, and reinforcing gradual progress toward these goals should help the client stay task- and goal-oriented.*

desirable task. They then have difficulty holding in their mind what they are supposed to be doing (working memory) and shifting away from (difficulties shifting responses) the activity they are distracted with back to the uninteresting task. They become wrapped up in the more desirable activity and suddenly have no sense of how much time they have lost. Due to the initial difficulty with inhibiting responses, they are now lost (on what they are supposed to be doing) and late (with completing the task in a timely manner). In this way, a client with ADHD can lose sight of their goal, especially long-term goals for speech fluency. If we consider the root of this whole spiral of problems to be in inhibiting responses, we can set up the session with minimal time for delay in the first place so that delay aversion is not triggered and therefore there are no more escape responses to inhibit. Keeping a "just right" pace in terms of interest and your client's ability to process, using visuals to remind your client of their short-term goals within the session, and reinforcing gradual progress toward these goals should help the client stay task and goal oriented.

*...it is so important to constantly check in with clients and, if working memory deficits are known or suspected, to provide as many written reminders of cues as possible.*

### Response Inhibition

Adults with ADHD-C have been shown to make more revisions in their speech, which investigators Engelhardt, Corley, Nigg, and Ferreira (2010) attribute to difficulties with the executive functioning skill of response inhibition. Anecdotally, many of my clients with cluttering (adults and children) report words coming out before they are ready. Preliminary findings from a replication of the Engelhardt et al. (2010) study in a small group of adults with cluttering have also found increased revisions to be a response pattern (Scaler Scott, Bossler, & Veneziale, 2015). Further study needs to be completed to determine whether difficulties with response inhibition are characteristic of all clients with ADHD and all clients with cluttering. However, if you have a client with cluttering and ADHD, it would stand to reason that difficulties with response inhibition may be more likely. In those cases, clients may benefit from use of pausing to give them increased formulation time. Although response inhibition has not yet been studied in those with atypical disfluency, due to frequent revisions in their speech and difficulties noted during formulation tasks, there is a potential link between response inhibition and atypical disfluency. Functionally, regardless of fluency diagnosis, if a client has multiple revisions, it can be a sign of difficulty with formulation, and use of increased pausing may be warranted.

### Self-Advocacy

If you are working with a client who is aware of their diagnosis of ADHD, it is a good idea to talk with them about what this diagnosis means. I think it goes without saying that if your client is a child, you would want to discuss this first with the client's caregiver. If permission is obtained, this talk should include the positives that have been found about the thinking of many with ADHD, the challenges ADHD brings to the client's daily life, and the strategies that work best for your client. Research literature has found specific strengths in the thinking patterns of those with ADHD, including creativity (White & Shah, 2006) and action orientation, making them strong candidates to become successful employees and entrepreneurs (Thurik, Khedhaouria, Torres, & Verheul, 2016). A document describing what ADHD is in laymen's terms is included at the end of this chapter. This document can be reviewed, discussed, and stored in a binder for future reference. Descriptions of fluency techniques (e.g., visual aids) can also be recorded in this binder. It is extremely important for a child to be aware of their learning style. As a child progresses in school, professionals working with them expect more and more for them to advocate for themselves. As a college professor, some of the best students I've had in my classes are not always those with the best grades. Instead, they are the students who know what things they need to do and ask for in order to succeed. If the clinician leaves an open door where clients can feel free to express opinions about how lessons are going and being perceived, this will help the client not only in fluency therapy but in other aspects of their lives where they need to self-advocate. Self-advocacy means explaining your learning strengths, challenges, and needs and making a plan to overcome your challenges. Self-advocacy does not mean making excuses for lapses in follow-through, but does mean helping others understand the root of these behaviors when they occur. As noted in the chapter on learning disabilities, a beneficial activity for the client would be to role-play educating the clinician (playing the role of "teacher") about their learning style, strengths, and needs. When ready, the client can practice using fluency strategies in this context just as they would in a real situation with a teacher or other professional.

### Medication

Finally, as many clients with ADHD may be taking some kind of medication, it is important to understand the potential effects of medication on behavioral performance and on fluency. For example, if your client with ADHD is scheduled to attend therapy first thing in the morning and is on a time-released medication, the medication may not have taken effect yet to ensure the most productive session. Likewise, medication could have worn off by the end of the day. It is important to discuss with caregivers the type(s) of medication(s) your client is taking and the peaks and valleys of when medications are thought to have the greatest impact. Realistically the client cannot always be scheduled in this optimal window, but when possible, it is ideal. Also of note are the findings that some psychostimulant medications used for ADHD can increase stuttering (see Healey & Reid, 2003, for review). As a clinician, you may be an important observer to any changes in a child's speech fluency in relation to changes in ADHD medications. The growing variety of medications available makes the relationship between newer medications and speech fluency unclear, and therefore the clinician's input all the more important.

# HOME PRACTICE AND CARRYOVER

Time management is a common area of struggle for our clients with attentional difficulties. Keep in mind that this will often affect whether or not your clients complete weekly assignments. It may be that your client does complete the assignment, but does not follow through with bringing the assignment to you. Or your client may forget altogether. In today's digital age, it is often helpful to get a client to complete an assignment in a way that is meaningful to them. For example, if you would like your client to keep a log of times they used their speech strategies, you may want to have them email or text as they complete a practice session rather than relying on paper and pencil. Not only may this be more motivating and meaningful for them, it also allows them to respond in the moment when they are thinking of it and it is fresh in their mind so they are less likely to forget. One thing to keep in mind with those with ADHD is that even though electronic devices work well, they only work well when they are charged and running. Kids with executive functioning deficits often don't plan ahead, leaving devices to run out of charge. Therefore, having another adult act as a "coach" to make sure that the client maintains these devices will help to ensure success.

In a similar manner, when assigned to practice strategies throughout the day, the client may often forget. It may be helpful to have the client choose the situations that are most meaningful, as these may stick better in their memory. For example, one client with ADHD and cluttering in our clinic was well-intentioned, but never completed paper logs of his fluency strategy practice. However, he said that several times a week he visited his local deli for lunch. He said that he often had to repeat himself due to unclear speech. We asked him to start ordering his lunch using his cluttering strategies and to notice any differences in responses from others. He did not write down what happened, but was excited to come back and tell us that in the past week, he had noticed that each time he ordered his lunch and used strategies, no one asked him to repeat himself, as they had in the past. It is moments like this, where clients can see meaningful change, that they are more likely to be motivated and remember to use strategies.

# CONCLUDING THOUGHTS

Included at the end of this chapter are activities reinforcing concepts discussed during this chapter and suggestions for using the positives of ADHD to harness success in your sessions (Table 8-1). Although this chapter has addressed many negative consequences of the brains of those with ADHD being wired differently, positive differences have also been found among those with ADHD. Those with ADHD have often been found to think outside the box and therefore are more likely to follow innovative career paths (Thurik et al., 2016). Given all the negative feedback a client may receive throughout their day, we should focus as much as possible on building success. I am a firm believer that if we understand where behaviors come from, we can structure our sessions for success.

| TABLE 8-1 |
|---|
| **Ways to Harness the Learning Styles of Clients With Attentional Challenges** |

| *LEARNING STYLE* | *STRATEGIES* |
|---|---|
| Seeks a fast pace | • Play fast-paced games<br>• Always remind client (but in a nonrushed way) to "keep it moving" when distracted by unrelated information<br>An example would be when a client is playing a game and before each turn has to practice a speech goal (e.g., use strategy at sentence level). Client is instructed to focus all energy on sentence then to switch focus to their turn in the game. In this way they keep both the practice and the game moving. |
| Can hyper-focus on areas of interest | • Use areas of interest as focus of speech topics |
| Is a creative thinker | • Have client develop the activity/activities for the session: goals, feedback<br>• Include content material on famous people with ADHD |
| Needs short-term rewards | • Build in rewards for goals within sessions |

# ACTIVITY 8-1:
# I WILL KEEP THIS IN MY MIND:
# EXTRA EFFORT SAVES ME TIME!

See if you can put in extra effort to get things right the first time. Then you won't have to do them again and you will save time!

Record some activities you did, your effort level in completing them, and how long they took you below. You can record your effort level as low, medium, or high. Remember, harder things or less interesting things will take more effort to keep focused.

| DATE | ACTIVITY | EFFORT LEVEL | DID I HAVE TO DO IT AGAIN? | HOW LONG DID THE WHOLE TASK TAKE (INCLUDING CORRECTIONS)? | HOW LONG DOES IT USUALLY TAKE? |
|------|----------|--------------|----------------------------|----------------------------------------------------------|--------------------------------|
|      |          |              |                            |                                                          |                                |
|      |          |              |                            |                                                          |                                |
|      |          |              |                            |                                                          |                                |
|      |          |              |                            |                                                          |                                |
|      |          |              |                            |                                                          |                                |
|      |          |              |                            |                                                          |                                |
|      |          |              |                            |                                                          |                                |
|      |          |              |                            |                                                          |                                |
|      |          |              |                            |                                                          |                                |
|      |          |              |                            |                                                          |                                |

# ACTIVITY 8-2:

**Student Activity:** Read the following information, and act out explaining this to your teacher, who will play the role of different teachers. Remember that some teachers may have a harder time than others understanding what ADHD is. You and your speech teacher can practice explaining these things to teachers who will understand quickly and others who will need more explanation.

## What Is Attention Deficit Hyperactivity Disorder?

It means that you have trouble focusing.

If you have ADHD, it does not mean you are not as smart as other people. In fact, a lot of famous people who have done great things have ADHD.

Research shows that people with ADHD create and invent lots of things that others without ADHD could not. This is because the brains of people with ADHD think about things differently. People with ADHD are very good at thinking outside the box.

## Is Attention Deficit Hyperactivity Disorder the Same Thing as Auditory Processing?

No. ADHD means someone gets distracted or can't focus. ADHD also means that you think differently or outside the box. Auditory processing is how your brain understands what you hear. Some people have trouble with auditory processing and have ADHD, but others have only one or the other.

## If You Have Trouble Paying Attention, Can That Affect How You Understand Something You Hear?

Yes. If someone is giving you directions and you are thinking about something else, it might be hard to understand the directions. If someone is giving you directions and something happens in the room that distracts you (like a noise), it might be hard to understand the directions.

# ACTIVITY 8-3:
# STRATEGY GAMES FOR FLUENCY PRACTICE

## Quick Practice Game With Preparatory Set

**Note**: Although we encourage parents not to rush children when speaking, there are times when school-aged children complain of wanting to interject an idea into a conversation with peers, blocking, and withdrawing from the conversation. To deal with this, I use the following activity to teach clients how to use a fluency strategy in a fast-paced situation. Additionally, although we may encourage gentle contacts and slowed speech, for many of our clients with ADHD, maintaining this in real situations may not be realistic for someone always feeling that they are driven by a motor. Therefore, teaching clients to use strategies effectively while not asking them to change who they are results in the best buy-in and carryover.

*Materials*: A deck of playing cards

*Directions*: Client and clinician play the card game "War" where each player puts a card out and the player with the highest card takes all of the cards. The object of the game is to collect all the cards.

*Incorporating the fluency strategy*: Client and clinician practice preparatory set while placing down cards:

**Client**: IIIIII am putting down an ace

**Clinician**: IIIII am putting down a 2

**Client**: IIIII win the card

## Speed Round

The goal of this round is to use the strategy before your opponent. You need to get the strategy out before your opponent does. You have to use the strategy while you are speaking. Being the first to say it doesn't make you win the round. You have to be the first to say it while using a strategy. Additionally, you have to be the first to use the strategy in an easy manner, that is, without tension.

**Note**: This helps clients learn a way to insert themselves into a conversation with friends when it is fast paced and everyone is talking quickly. Often in these times, if the client tries to insert themselves, they may become stuck. But if they use a strategy proactively and quickly, it will help them contribute to this conversation.

**Client**: IIIII have a 2

**Clinician**: IIIII have an ace

**Client** (says it first): IIII steal your card

If clinician was first to say "IIII win the card," they would get it. But if the client is first to use the strategy, they get to steal the card, even though their card is the lower number.

# ACTIVITY 8-4:
# YOU BE THE SPEECH TEACHER!

**Directions:** Work with your speech teacher to set your goals for today's session and over a longer period of time.

## Long-Term Goals:

- What are my goals for speech when I am done?


- Is there a reward I am working toward? What is it? How do I earn it?


## Short-Term Goals:

- What is my goal for today's speech session? Be specific.


- Example: I will say 10 sentences with prep set correctly.


- What activity would I like to use to work on my goal?


- How will I work my goal into this activity?


- Is there a reward I am working toward for today's goal? What is it? How do I earn it?

# CHAPTER 9

# Autism Spectrum Disorder

## Definitions

The diagnostic criteria for autism spectrum disorder (ASD) was recently redefined in the *Diagnostic and Statistical Manual of Mental Disorders, Fifth Edition* (DSM-5; American Psychiatric Association, 2013). For a diagnosis of autism, clients must demonstrate deficits in the areas of social communication and interaction across a variety of contexts, as well as repetitive or restrictive patterns of behavior. Severity of autism ranges from level 1, requiring support; to level 2, requiring "substantial" support; to level 3, requiring "very substantial support." After it has been determined that they meet the diagnostic criteria for autism and have been assessed for severity level, those with autism are determined to present with or without intellectual impairment and with or without language impairment (American Psychiatric Association, 2013). Although some may be diagnosed without language impairment, it is important to keep in mind how the language impairment (or lack thereof) is defined. For example, by the definition in the DSM-5, if language impairment were to include social pragmatic difficulties, then 100% of those diagnosed with ASD would have an accompanying language impairment. If language impairment were defined by only difficulties with semantics or syntax, then not all with ASD would have language impairment. Additionally, the definition of a language impairment may include only those identified by standardized tests, or it may include both those identified by standardized measures and by authentic language/discourse samples. If it is defined by standardized measures only, then not all with autism will present with a language impairment. But if it is also defined by difficulties with discourse, then nearly—if not all—with autism could be considered to present with a language impairment (Hale & Tager-Flusberg, 2005). Often a client is diagnosed with ASD by a neurodevelopmental pediatrician, psychologist, neuropsychologist, or psychiatrist. When you begin working with a client who has received the diagnosis of autism, I advise you to use your clinical judgment about whether intervention and goals are required in the area of language.

Scaler Scott, K.
*Fluency Plus: Managing Fluency Disorders in Individuals With Multiple Diagnoses (pp 143-159).*
© 2018 Taylor & Francis Group.

# WHAT FLUENCY DISORDERS ARE FOUND IN THIS POPULATION?

All fluency disorders have been found in individuals with ASD. These fluency disorders have been identified in all levels of autism, including those with and without intellectual disability (see Scaler Scott, Tetnowski, Flaitz, & Yaruss, 2014, for review; Scaler Scott, 2011). Those with ASD have been found to present with stuttering characterized by affective, cognitive, and behavioral components, as well as secondary behaviors and avoidance (Scaler Scott et al., 2014). Cluttering has also been found in the ASD population (Scaler Scott et al., 2014). Atypical disfluency has been found in school-aged children (Scaler Scott et al., 2014), teens (Scaler Scott, Grossman, Abendroth, Tetnowski, & Damico, 2007; Sisskin, 2006), and preschool children (Plexico, Cleary, McAlpine, & Plumb, 2010) with ASD (see Sisskin & Wasilus, 2014, for review).

Although everyone with ASD does not have a fluency disorder in terms of fluency of speech, many with ASD have a difficult time getting their message across fluently from a language perspective (Ochs & Solomon, 2004). This is often due to difficulties with verbal organization and may result in multiple revisions. Lake, Humphreys, and Cardy (2011) found that those on the autism spectrum use fewer filled pauses than those without ASD. That is, the study participants with autism didn't use words such as "um," "uh," or other fillers to let the listener know they are still organizing thoughts or trying to think of a word. These are called listener-oriented strategies (Lake et al., 2011). The participants in the study with ASD tended to use more speaker-oriented strategies, such as placing long pauses while they were thinking of words (Lake et al., 2011). In daily situations, these pauses may be misinterpreted by the listener, and the speaker with ASD may be interrupted and become frustrated. In addition to long pauses, investigators have theorized that because those with autism have difficulty with perspective taking and theory of mind (both related to the ability to understand the listener's needs), they may leave out necessary background information, provide irrelevant details, and/or fail to provide enough pronoun referents in their discourse (Colle, Baron-Cohen, Wheelwright, & van der Lely, 2008). This gives the impression of incohesive, disorganized discourse. Whether the discourse difficulties stem from perspective taking, theory of mind, or other issues related to understanding listener needs, those with autism have been found to struggle with getting a message across fluently, even if their speech is otherwise fluent.

*All fluency disorders have been found in individuals with ASD.*

*Although everyone with ASD does not have a fluency disorder in terms of fluency of speech, many with ASD have a difficult time getting their message across fluently from a language perspective (Ochs & Solomon, 2004).*

# MYTHS AND FACTS REGARDING FLUENCY TREATMENT IN AUTISM SPECTRUM DISORDER

One myth is that those with autism are unaware of their difficulties with fluency and therefore not bothered by them. Given difficulties those with ASD have with self-monitoring, this may be true in a larger percentage of cases than in those without autism. However, to date, this theory has not been tested. Additionally, there are individuals with autism who present with affective and/or cognitive components of fluency disorders. Therefore, not all are lacking in awareness, and not all are unaffected by their issues with fluency.

Another myth is that because those with autism have so many other goals to work on, fluency should be the last priority. This should be assessed on an individual basis. If fluency issues are leading to communication avoidance, then certainly no progress in language or pragmatics can be made without addressing the fluency. A third myth is that disfluency does not contribute negatively to social interaction. Although in theory all peers should be patient listeners, research has shown that as early as pre-school years, peers may choose

*There are individuals with autism who present with affective and/or cognitive components of fluency disorders. Therefore, not all are lacking in awareness, and not all unaffected by their issues with fluency.*

to spend less time with a child with a communication impairment (Gertner, Rice, & Hadley, 1994). If, for example, a client has difficulty expressing himself or herself clearly due to multiple revisions, this may result in peers not engaging them in conversation. In cases such as these, work on fluency will also enhance social interaction.

I am not suggesting that a client with autism needs to decrease stuttering for their listener's efficiency. What I am suggesting is that some with ASD may have difficulty focusing on the main points and/or get bogged down in details and/or revise utterances to find just the right wording, making it difficult for their listener to understand them. These are areas that are important to address whether they are rooted in fluency, language, or pragmatic issues. The bottom line is that the client needs to understand what their listener needs in order to process their message. In the case of clients with ASD, fluency treatment may not be about expecting clients to be completely fluent at all times, but about managing moments of stuttering, cluttering, atypical disfluency, and/or excessive disfluency so that they can communicate as efficiently as possible. Efficiency does not mean that we wish our clients to over-simplify their message. Without sacrificing their main point or content, we need to help the client get to the point as efficiently as possible. That being said, something to keep in mind is that although there is no current research on this topic, when I have asked some of my clients with autism whether they are telling a story just to hear it again or for the listener to understand, they do say that the retelling is not always for the listener. This is important to keep in mind because if the client is telling the story just to hear it, they may be resistant to make the story more efficient or understandable for their listener. Typically, though, I find that a certain percentage of the time, the client does want the listener to understand the message they are conveying. I focus on these times to help the client gain perspective on why using strategies to make their speech more efficient will help their listener process their message.

It may be the case that disfluency is not negatively interfering with communication and that the client has other goals to work on that are higher priority. This is fine, as long as fluency is monitored and revisited when the timing is right. For example, if suddenly communication avoidance should increase, then the fluency disorder that was once put on the back burner may need to be prioritized. If a client getting their message across is interfering with conversation skills with others and/or academic or work performance, then treatment focusing on the relevant fluency disorder leading to this difficulty (i.e., stuttering, cluttering, excessive disfluency, and/or atypical disfluency) should be prioritized. When fluency treatment is prioritized, then strategies to help get the client through difficult moments of communication can be taught. When the client gains some skill with these strategies, they can begin to incorporate these strategies into other tasks in therapy sessions, such as language-related tasks.

# What Executive Functioning Issues Can I Expect in Autism Spectrum Disorder?

Although not an executive functioning (EF) deficit, sensory sensitivities in clients with autism are something that bear mentioning before the discussion of executive functions, as they can have a negative impact upon EF skills. One potential symptom that may contribute to the diagnosis of autism according to the DSM-5 criteria is over-reactivity or under-reactivity to sensory stimuli in the environment (American Psychiatric Association, 2013). If a client is over-reactive to stimuli, they may find certain lights, sounds, tastes, or textures more aversive than most people without sensory sensitivity would. If they are underreactive to stimuli, they may not notice pain in the same way that others would. For example, they may not realize that a stove is hot and burning their hand until it is too late. How this may apply to your session is that these clients who are underreactive are often known as "sensory seekers." They will seek out a sensation to meet a sensory need. If a child is a sensory seeker and needs more feedback than the average person from their hand, they may pound their fist on the table. At first glance this may seem like a behavior issue. But if the client has known sensory issues, it may be viewed in a different light. People do not have to be diagnosed with autism to have sensory issues. However, sensory issues are quite common in autism (see Stewart et al., 2015, for review). Next we will examine how these sensory sensitivities can contribute to EF deficits. If you need more information about a client's sensory profile, you should consult with a licensed occupational therapist experienced in the area of sensory integration.

*EF deficits are proposed by some autism researchers as a core issue in ASD (Ozonoff, Pennington, & Rogers, 1991).*

EF deficits are proposed by some autism researchers as a core issue in ASD (Ozonoff et al., 1991). Issues the clinician may expect to see include all areas discussed in Chapter 4 of this book: attention to task, self-awareness and self-monitoring, goal setting, inhibiting responses, retrieval, working memory, phonological encoding, cognitive flexibility, problem solving, and task persistence. Although each of these areas has been identified in one or more studies of autism, findings are inconsistent between studies. For example, the literature on response inhibition does not always show deficits in autism for inhibiting response related to behavior, but does show difficulties with response inhibition when related to visual tasks (Agam, Joseph, Barton, & Manoach, 2010). The literature on working memory also does not show deficits consistently. Some investigators believe that these deficits may exist, but that the difficulties may be secondary to deficits in other areas. For example, the complex information-processing model of ASD states that weaknesses will vary with the demands of the task and with the level of deficits the client has in terms of sensory processing, motor and memory impairments, and difficulties with expressive language. (Minshew & Williams, 2008). This model proposes that if you follow two individuals with autism with a similar cognitive profile, their ability to each process information from the environment will depend on the load that the situation places upon their system and the weakest areas for each client. For example, if one of these clients has severe sensitivity to noise and both clients are placed in a situation with increased background noise, it stands to reason that the client who is more sensitive to noise will likely process less information than the second. It is not that the one client necessarily has more impaired auditory processing, but that the processing difficulties in this client are secondary to the sensory difficulties. Therefore, the sensory sensitivities place more load on this client's system. If a client has severe difficulties processing sensory information in general, their system will be more taxed, and more difficulties in the areas of EF may present themselves. However, when the client's environment is well controlled, these same EF deficits will not necessarily occur. The bottom line here is that performance depends on the demands on the client's system and what the client's system can handle in each of the areas before the system is "taxed." This explains why studies of isolated EF tasks do not always capture the difficulties in autism that are reported by caregivers in everyday tasks. Likewise, difficulties with fluency of speech may not always present themselves in out-of-context testing, but may be noted more in the context of everyday speech.

From a practical standpoint, whether you subscribe to the view that EF deficits represent a core deficit area in autism or whether you feel other issues result in EF deficits, the best service you can do your clients is to 1) be aware of the EF deficits a client may have and 2) study what behaviors precede difficulties in EF that get in the way of therapy progress. For example, if your client seems to be having difficulties with attention, notice what precedes these difficulties. Is it that your client is frustrated and having a difficult time communicating to you why, so they are using distraction as an escape from the frustration? In this case, the root issue would be problem solving the frustration. You would need to work with them on how to communicate that they are frustrated. Additionally, you might study the frustration reaction to see what precedes this so that if appropriate, you can modify tasks accordingly. Does your client have attention difficulties with other professionals or just you? If it is just you, is it related to their sensory sensitivity to a perfume you wear that can be taxing their ability to attend? Is their difficulty with attention related to the task and past negative experiences with it? We had a client in our university clinic who found practicing connecting his words for continuous phonation very aversive. When we asked the caregivers about this reaction and whether he'd always had it, they noted that it began in school when a speech teacher was quite tough on using continuous phonation. In this case, his past negative experiences combined with decreased task persistence for difficult tasks resulted in his noncompliance. We went with the theory that the task had negative association for him, but also that it was too difficult (he was not really connecting what the clinician wanted him to do). We decided instead to change our approach and use preparatory set (described as rainbow speech in Chapters 5 and 6). This is an example of how we needed to observe the behavior, formulate hypotheses about it, test the hypotheses, and change the situation to make the session more successful. Another example occurred with one of my clients on the autism spectrum who exhibited word-final disfluencies. I was working with him on pausing to give himself formulation time. When we first began this task at the structured sentence level, he had no problem with it. When asked to pause in connected speech, he became resistant. He often did not respond to cues to use pauses, but instead kept talking. Sometimes if he didn't respond to a nonverbal signal, I gave a verbal reminder: "Remember to pause." It was during one of these moments when he became very frustrated, stopped his story, and said, "That's why I hate pausing. Then people interrupt you and you forget what you're going to say." He saw the cue for pausing as an interruption. He was worried that someone would interrupt verbally and he would lose his train of thought. He hadn't been able to verbalize this thought until right in the moment of losing his train of thought. Had such a moment not occurred, I could have taken his lack of response to my cues as noncompliance. Certainly his resistance reflected some inflexibility, but that inflexibility was likely rooted in difficulties problem solving. When we realized what the problem was, we were able to teach him strategies to help him hold his thought in his mind. In this way, he was better equipped to handle using pausing and potential "interruptions" in conversation, should his listener need to stop him to make a comment, ask a question, etc.

Even if EF deficits exist in isolation, their implications often are most apparent in contextualized activities. For example, although a client may be able to use fluency strategies in a structured session, when speaking on a topic about which they are very knowledgeable and/or interested, and/or in a high-stress social situation, they may not be able to use their strategies. Their working memory may be too taxed by demands to formulate the message and/or to engage in appropriate social interaction for them to be able to also access fluency strategies. It should be kept in mind that the client's ability to use strategies will vary by situation and/or speaking context. The various EF components of the system that could be challenged should be kept in mind whenever working with a client with ASD. In this way, the clinician can get to the root of what is likely getting in the way of progress and either work directly on that area (if applicable) or provide compensatory strategies to assist with the problem area.

# MANAGING EXECUTIVE FUNCTIONING DEFICITS

## Letting Perseveration Be Your Friend

Many with ASD have focused interests. Some would consider these to be fixations. Some would say not to engage the client in their fixations for topics of conversation, except maybe initially during evaluation. After all, we work on pragmatic language, right? Isn't it our job to teach clients that everyone may not want to hear about ceiling fans and vacuum cleaners? Although I understand the value of these statements, I feel that a balance can be achieved. For fluency therapy, we want to get our clients talking as much as possible. The more they talk, the more they have opportunities to practice managing moments of disfluency. Our clients already have difficulty thinking of what to talk about outside of these interests. Should we broaden their horizons? Yes, of course. But perhaps we can broaden them in other aspects of therapy. For fluency therapy, we can let them know that this is a good time to talk about topics of interest. We can ask questions and let them know that we appreciate them teaching us all there is to know about the topic. This makes our clients feel that their message has value (Scaler Scott & Ward, 2013). For some with ASD, knowing that you care about what they are saying can be very valuable. At the end of an evaluation, one of my clients with ASD said, "Thank you for listening to me. Most people don't want to hear all I know about dinosaurs." I not only learned more about dinosaurs, but I got the nice long language sample I wanted and needed to observe the client's disfluency.

> *Even if EF deficits exist in isolation, they often are seen in contextualized activities.*

## An Important Note About Self-Awareness, Communication Attitudes, and Choosing a Therapy Approach

You may work with clients with ASD who can benefit from direct feedback about changing their speech with little concern for negative communication attitudes. For example, the young man who worked on fluency rules in the Brundage, Whelan, and Burgess (2013) study was reported to benefit from such rules as "say a word only once." For those without ASD, this type of cue might raise a feeling of shame in a client who wants to follow the rule but finds she or he cannot. In some with ASD, they do not seem to be sensitive to their disfluency and working on it in such a rule-based manner. The rule-based manner fits with the learning styles of many with ASD. That being said, I have also worked with many clients with ASD who are very sensitive to cues to change their speech. If this is the case, you should investigate the root cause of the resistance so that you can treat it accordingly. For example, recall my client who was resistant to cues to pause due to thinking that he would lose his train of thought. Others may not be keen on changing their speech as they have difficulties with cognitive flexibility, making it difficult for them to adapt to a new speaking pattern. When getting to know a new client with ASD, the clinician should

> *You may work with clients with ASD who can benefit from direct feedback about changing their speech with little concern for negative communication attitudes.*

watch the client's reactions to cues for direct speech change. Recall that the clinician should look for what happens right before a client's response to determine the root of the reaction. This will help you plan accordingly for future delivery of cues. You will need to use your clinical judgment about whether the client will benefit from a rule-based approach or become too frustrated with it.

As most practicing clinicians are likely aware, it has been documented that the brains of those with autism function differently from those of neurotypicals. This was found in some of the recent literature on EF. Researchers found that those with autism didn't use words (as neurotypical controls did) to help them navigate difficulties with working memory (Joseph, Steele, Meyer, & Tager-Flusberg, 2005). In another study, investigators also found that under functional magnetic resonance imaging conditions, adults with high-functioning autism showed more brain activation in regions suggesting use of visual codes to complete a working memory task, whereas controls showed more brain activation in areas suggesting use of verbal codes for task completion (Koshino, Carpenter, Minshew, Cherkassky, Keller, & Just, 2005). Based upon these findings and the literature that outlines differences in cognitive processes in autism vs. controls (Constable, Ring, Bowler, & Gaigg, 2017), I choose to use visualization as a working memory strategy rather than verbal rehearsal. How does addressing working memory relate to fluency work? If we are trying to get our clients to use pausing to help with fluency (very often in cluttering and/or atypical disfluency) and they are afraid that pausing will result in them forgetting their message, we need to help solve the memory issue. Therefore, I teach pausing combined with visualization to assist clients with holding information in memory.

Of late, I have been working with clients with autism level 1 who are very insightful about how they think. They have been verbal about how they feel a certain strategy may not work for their thinking process. For example, I tend to use a linear visual organizer to help clients organize verbal information. I have had some clients with ASD tell me that they do not find this type of organizer helpful, as they think in a different manner. When this is the case, I give clients a choice of several types of organizers and let them choose the ones that resonate the most with their learning style. Likewise, I also use the concept of different types of minds to help my clients understand when they may need to shift the way in which they present information to accommodate their listener's learning style. For example, perhaps they enjoy telling a story in extreme detail. We talk about good and not-so-good times to do this. We also talk about how certain listeners (such as caregivers) may be able to process these details, whereas other listeners (such as teachers or peers) may need only the main points to understand, as they may have difficulty pulling the main points out on their own. I liken this to adjustments a speaker makes to their speech when they need to shorten and/or simplify language for young children. In having open discussions with clients about the reasons for strategies as well as trying to honor what resonates best with them, I get the most buy-in to long-term strategy use.

*...it has been documented that the brains of those with autism function differently from those of neurotypicals...*

The following activities focus on fluency practice in the context of understanding the learning style of autism. Often I use these activities both to reinforce fluency practice and to provide continued practice in other communication areas that may be needed by someone with autism. Table 9-1 summarizes ways to incorporate fluency work in conjunction with work on specific EF needs.

| TABLE 9-1 | | |
|---|---|---|
| **Ideas for Relevant Activities Related to Fluency Goals and Specific Areas of Executive Functioning** | | |
| *EXECUTIVE FUNCTIONING SKILL* | *ACTIVITIES TO TARGET* | *WAYS TO INCORPORATE STRATEGY PRACTICE FOR STUTTERING, CLUTTERING, ATYPICAL DISFLUENCY, EXCESSIVE NON–STUTTERING-LIKE DISFLUENCIES* |
| Cognitive flexibility | Generating multiple solutions to speaking problems | Use strategies while speaking in games, when talking about solutions to problems. Follow speech hierarchy: <br> • Words <br> • Phrases <br> • Sentences <br> • Reading <br> • Structured conversation <br> • Unstructured conversation |
| Working memory | Any memory game that involves using visualizing while speaking or listening | |
| Retrieval | Activities requiring categorization, generating synonyms, antonyms | |
| Response inhibition | Activities that require the speaker to filter distractions while speaking | |
| Self-monitoring | Activities that require monitoring their own speech and/or the speech of others | |

# ACTIVITY 9-1:
# PERSPECTIVE-TAKING ACTIVITY FOR CLUTTERING

## *What Is Cluttering?*

Cluttering is a speech disorder where the listener has a hard time understanding you. It often happens when someone speaks quickly.

## *Why Should I Care About Cluttering?*

When someone clutters, the listener may not understand them. If you want the person you are talking with to understand you and not become confused, you should try to use as clear speech as possible. For example, if you ask someone for a bottle of cranapple juice and they think you say "apple juice," you might not get what you requested. It may be frustrating for you if others don't understand you and ask you to repeat yourself a lot.

## *How Will the Listener Feel If They Don't Understand Me?*

They may feel confused or frustrated.

## *What Will the Listener Do If They Don't Understand Me?*

It depends on the listener. Some will ask you to repeat as many times as needed to understand. Some may ask you to repeat yourself only once. If they still don't understand you, they may just try and figure out what they think you are saying and respond to that. Sometimes they may guess correctly, but many times they will not.

## *Shouldn't the Listener Always Ask to Be Sure They Understand Me?*

This may be true. But it doesn't always happen. Sometimes listeners think they will make you uncomfortable if they ask you too many times. Maybe you've gotten frustrated with them in the past. So sometimes they just try to do their best to figure out what you might mean. If you know the listener well and have a good relationship with them, you can tell them if you want them to ask you to repeat until they get your message. You just have to try your best not to get frustrated with their requests!

## *Activity*

**Directions:** Use your fluency strategies while talking with your speech clinician about the two scenes below.

Pretend I am your good friend. Tell me about cluttering and what you'd like me to do as a listener.

Now pretend I am an adult you don't know very well. You just met me—I am a friend of your parents. Tell why it would be important to use your cluttering strategies to speak as clearly as you can to me.

# ACTIVITY 9-2:
# PROBLEM-SOLVING ACTIVITY FOR
# CLUTTERING, ATYPICAL DISFLUENCY, OR
# EXCESSIVE NON–STUTTERING-LIKE DISFLUENCIES

**Directions**: When solving the problems below, use fluency strategies as instructed by your speech teacher. Your speech teacher may ask you to write out answers first, then share them orally using your strategies. In parentheses after each problem are notes for your speech teacher.

**Problem One**:
You notice that when your friend is telling you a story, they keep changing the wording of what they say. List two reasons this could be (EF skills addressed: generating multiple causes to problem situations, cognitive flexibility).

1.

2.

**Problem Two**:
You are talking with someone and you hear lots of filler words in your speech. Name two solutions you can try to decrease filler words (EF skills addressed: generating multiple solutions, cognitive flexibility).

1.

2.

**Problem Three:**

You are telling a story and all of a sudden feel lost and can't remember what point you were making. What are two things you could do to help get you back on track (EF skills addressed: generating multiple solutions, cognitive flexibility)?

1.



2.

# ACTIVITY 9-3:
# DON'T SAY IT! AN ACTIVITY FOR
# INHIBITING RESPONSES AND STUTTERING

**Directions**: Play a guessing game where you and your opponent take turns giving each other clues about something in the room. Don't guess the object until you are absolutely certain. Keep thinking silently about each new clue, trying to put all of the clues together. Points are scored for each guess you make, and the person with the lowest score wins.

When you ask for another clue or guess, use cancellation, pullout, or preparatory set to make your guess. Examples:

C—an (pause after finishing word) Caaan you give me another clue? (cancellation)

I—(pause after block and finishing word) IIIII am going to guess the chair. (cancellation)

C-c-c-c-aaaan you give another clue? (pullout)

I-I-I-I-IIIIIII am going to guess the chair. (pullout)

Caaan you give me another clue? (preparatory set)

IIIII am going to guess the chair. (preparatory set)

# ACTIVITY 9-4:
# CAN YOU GIVE ME ANOTHER CLUE? AN ACTIVITY FOR COGNITIVE FLEXIBILITY AND RETRIEVAL

**Directions**: You will choose an object for your opponent to guess. Your opponent will ask for more clues as needed. They will say, "Can you give me another clue?" Your job is to think of as many clues as possible. Use a stuttering strategy when you give each clue, as instructed by your speech teacher.

**Examples**:

The f—irst (pause after block and completion of word) fiiirst clue is that it is round. (cancellation)

The second c-c-c-luuuuue is that it is red. (pullout)

The next clue iiiiis that it is crunchy. (preparatory set)

Jot some ideas for objects in the space below:

# ACTIVITY 9-5:
# TAKE A PICTURE AND DON'T LOSE IT!
# A WORKING MEMORY GAME

**Directions**: You and your opponent will take turns making up a story and adding to it. Try to visualize the story in your mind and make that visualization change each time something is added to the story. This will help you be able to tell the story without forgetting it. Use speech strategies as instructed by your speech reacher while you are telling your story.

**Hint**: It often helps to picture each part of your story like a scene in a movie. You can describe each scene to your listener as if you are describing scenes in a movie.

Here's an example: // = pause

First//the kids are all in the kitchen eating dinner.// Then next//they get up to go into the living room.// In the living room//they talk about what games to play.// Mary goes into the game closet//and comes back with three games.

Use the space below to keep track of any points for telling the story. Points can be awarded for use of speech strategies, adding new details to the story, whatever your speech teacher decides!

# ACTIVITY 9-6:
# HOW WELL AM I DOING? HOW WELL DID I DO?
## AN ACTIVITY FOR SELF-MONITORING

**Directions for home assignment part 1**: Notice where people put "ums" or "uhs" in their speech. These are good places for pauses. Can you monitor your mom, dad, speech teacher, or other adult and remind them of good places for pauses? Tell your speech teacher about how it went. Your speech teacher may have you jot some notes below, then tell about it using your speech strategies.

**Directions for home assignment part 2**: After you have completed part 1 above, listen for what signs you hear that the speaker is getting confused about how to say something. What do they do? Check any things you noticed below.

☐ Saying "um" or "uh"

☐ Repeating a phrase over and over (I want to, I want to, I want to go)

☐ Changing what they are saying a lot (I want some tea, no cof-, wait, maybe I'll have soda)

Listen for these signs in yourself. Is this a good place for pausing?

Tell your speech teacher about how it went. Your speech teacher may have you jot some notes below, then tell about it using your speech strategies.

# ACTIVITY 9-7:
# BEING SOMEONE ELSE'S BRAIN

**Directions**: This activity will help you to ignore distractions in your mind. All players will brainstorm topics that they get distracted by in their minds. List the topics in the table below.

| PLAYER NAME | DISTRACTING TOPICS |
|---|---|
|  |  |
|  |  |
|  |  |
|  |  |
|  |  |

Once the table is complete, take turns telling each other stories. As one person is telling a story, the listener is pretending to be the speaker's brain by randomly making short comments about the speaker's distracting topics (e.g., "Boy I am really hungry").

The speaker earns points for:

- Ignoring these distractions

- Staying with the story

# ACTIVITY 9-8:
## RULES FOR CONVERSATION

To the speech clinician: The rules below address many of the areas I find are lacking in clients who present with atypical disfluencies. Each of these rules can be made into its own activity, or, once understood by the client, reinforced in other activities involving spontaneous speech.

## *Things to Remember When Having a Conversation*

1. When you are asked a question, try to answer the question and not something else!

2. When you are asked a question, try to focus on the big picture unless the other person asks you for more details.

3. When you are telling the other person something, try to stay focused to what you are saying. Ignore distractions. Distractions can be:

   **Internal**: Means inside your mind, like while you are talking about something, all of the sudden your mind thinks of something else.

   **External**: Means outside of yourself, like while you are talking about something, all of the sudden someone or something makes a noise, or interrupts you

4. Be sure to use pauses. Pauses will help your listener have time to follow your message because the pauses will slow you down a little.

5. Stay on the main topic of conversation. Don't switch to another topic at random times.

6. Keep your eyes on the person you are talking with and your hands and body still.

7. If all your focus is on the conversation and the person you are talking with, this is called being engaged with the other person.

# CHAPTER 10

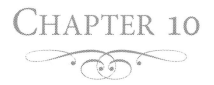

# SELECTIVE MUTISM

## DEFINITION

Selective mutism (SM) is a disorder whereby the client exhibits normal communication in select situations (such as in a home environment) but exhibits limited communication in other situations (such as at school). The origins of SM are thought to be based in anxiety disorders (American Psychiatric Association, 2013). You may be asking yourself, why would a speech-language clinician be involved in treatment of someone with an anxiety disorder? Although this disorder is based in anxiety, it results in difficulties with daily communication. For example, I have worked with cases where the child has such difficulty communicating in their school environment that they will have an accident rather than ask to go to the bathroom. Because the symptoms we are treating are related to communication, we are the communication experts who can help with determining functional communication strategies while anxiety is being addressed. For example, while a child is working on becoming comfortable speaking more in their classroom environment, they still need to be able to communicate daily needs such as going to the bathroom. The clinician can provide suggestions for alternative means of communicating, such as a nonverbal signal or using some type of low-tech communication board. Additionally, the speech-language clinician is skilled at working on communication in hierarchical steps. Therefore, the clinician can design a program of helping the client approach more and more difficult communication situations. The speech-language clinician is the most logical professional to determine a hierarchy that progresses in a logical order and that considers the speech, language, and pragmatic demands of each situation in the hierarchy. In general, the treatment of SM involves treatment of communication by speech-language clinicians. That being said, because the root of SM is anxiety, treatment works best when the clinician works in conjunction with a licensed psychologist, psychiatrist, or counselor.

Scaler Scott, K.
*Fluency Plus: Managing Fluency Disorders in
Individuals With Multiple Diagnoses (pp 161-173).*
© 2018 Taylor & Francis Group.

# MYTHS AND FACTS REGARDING SELECTIVE MUTISM

The first myth is inherent to the name of the disorder. Those with SM are not mute. By definition, those with SM have normal communication in selected (hence the name) situations; therefore, they are not mute. In selected other situations, they may, in fact, be mute and not communicating verbally at all. That brings us to the next myth. A client does not have to be completely mute in these situations to be diagnosed with SM. Often they do speak somewhat, just significantly less than in other situations. I have seen children who have been determined not to qualify for a diagnosis of SM because they are not completely mute. In these situations, the child's limited use of speech in selected situations has been described as "just being shy." Shyness is not the issue here. If there is a question whether the diagnosis is appropriate, remember that the speech-language clinician is not the one who would make the diagnosis. It is important to refer the client to a psychologist who has specific experience with diagnosing SM. Accurate diagnosis helps to ensure accurate treatment.

*A client does not have to be completely mute to be diagnosed with SM.*

In its pure form, SM occurs without a communication disorder. However, because clients with SM can also have a coexisting communication disorder, they should be carefully assessed by the speech-language clinician. Obtaining language samples from caregivers in situations where the client speaks more freely will be extremely valuable in completing an accurate assessment. Keep in mind that if the client does experience anxiety, any testing situation and/or situation with an unfamiliar listener such as a speech-language clinician may result in decreased communication. It is difficult to complete an accurate assessment of a client's expressive language when the client is inhibited during the evaluation session. Therefore, any receptive tests that require pointing may be a good place to start in assessing for a potential communication disorder. The assessment may need to be ongoing, where new data are compiled as rapport develops between client and clinician. Although extra time may be needed, it is critical for the clinician to gain an accurate picture of the client's profile, including any communication difficulties, so that the most appropriate treatment plan can be developed.

Another set of myths relates to interpretation of the behaviors of someone with SM. Because, like fluency disorders, SM does not occur in all contexts, this may cause some who interact with your client to question whether or not they really can communicate easily and are not just "faking it" in certain settings. Some may misinterpret lack of communication as a form of purposeful manipulation to gain attention, get out of work, etc. This is not the case. When someone has a diagnosis of SM, their root problem is based in anxiety, not behavior. Additionally, when communicating with someone with SM, you may note that they seem to present with flat affect. Some have commented about this look as a face that is "blank" or "mask-like." This might make you question pragmatic skills. Of course, it is possible the client could have a concomitant pragmatic diagnosis. But it is very important to distinguish between a pragmatic deficit and someone who has anxiety. Anxiety can result in the mask-like face when communicating with others. Those with just SM are not lacking in knowledge of social rules or perspective taking. In fact, if you either observe the client in environments where they do speak more freely or view recordings

*...because clients with SM can also have a coexisting communication disorder, they should be carefully assessed by the speech-language clinician.*

of these situations, you will likely see that pragmatic language skills are intact. Someone with a pragmatic language deficit might not talk to another person and not realize that this is uncomfortable for their listener. On the other hand, someone with SM might not talk, know it is uncomfortable, and want to communicate in a regular manner, but because of anxiety, be unable to do so.

It is really important for the clinician and all professionals working with the client to know that because the lack of talking is not based in a behavior issue, positive reinforcement of verbal responses will not work. This is important to consider as the client begins to progress in therapy and becomes more verbal. Understanding this concept about SM will help the speech-language clinician to advocate on behalf of the child. It is intuitive for a teacher, parent, or other professional to praise someone's attempts at talking when they see them. However, for someone with SM, this praise can result in regression rather than progression. Those with SM often do not like being the center of attention, and anything that puts them in this position may cause them to become anxious and stop communicating (Dummit, Klein, Tancer, Asche, Martin, & Fairbanks, 1997). When a client with SM begins to increase their verbal communication, communication partners should respond as they would to any other speaker rather than with praise, surprise, and/or excitement.

> *When someone has a diagnosis of SM, their root problem is based in anxiety, not behavior.*

## FLUENCY DISORDERS FOUND IN SELECTIVE MUTISM

You may be thinking that this doesn't sound like a child who will talk that much; therefore, how could they possibly exhibit fluency concerns? Remember that in selected situations, the client will speak normally or, if they have a communication impairment, at least to their "normal" level. Co-occurrence of stuttering and/or cluttering in family members of those with SM has been documented (Viana, Beidel, & Rabian, 2009). At times when fluency disorders co-occur with SM, it is difficult to know whether the SM may have developed out of anxiety secondary to sensitivity to the fluency disorder. This is not to say that disfluency causes SM. There is no evidence to support such a causal link. However, it is possible that if someone is prone to SM, difficult events such as stuttering may trigger SM symptoms. For example, we had a client in our clinic whose SM was found to be triggered by a traumatic event at her school. The event involved negative listener reaction to her stuttering. Therefore, the outward manifestation of her SM symptoms was intertwined with negative feelings about stuttering and communication. Although it is not yet documented in the literature, there is no reason to believe that atypical disfluency or cluttering couldn't co-occur with SM. As of this writing, I have treated one case where the client presented with SM and word-final disfluencies (WFDs). As I conducted an assessment over time, I was able to learn from the assessment and from her mother's report that the anxiety seemed to come from SM alone, as the client was unaware of her WFDs.

> *Those with SM often do not like being the center of attention, and anything that puts them in this position may cause them to become anxious and stop communicating*

Given the fact that receptive and expressive language disorders can co-occur with SM (Hua & Major, 2016; McInnes, Fung, Manassis, Fiksenbaum, & Tannock, 2004), it is also reasonable to see excessive non–stuttering-like disfluencies (NSLDs) in those with SM related to an expressive language disorder.

## EXECUTIVE FUNCTIONING ISSUES IN SELECTIVE MUTISM

Currently there are no studies documenting executive functioning (EF) difficulties in those with SM. Of course, it is possible that those with SM can have other diagnoses such as attention deficit hyperactivity disorder, in which case the EF issues the clinician might expect can be found in the relevant chapters of this book for each diagnosis. Although there are no known EF issues in SM, it is highly possible that anxiety from SM may have an impact upon other EF issues. For example, when someone is anxious, whether they have SM or not,

*Those with just SM are not lacking in knowledge of social rules or perspective taking (Dummit, Klein, Tancer, Asche, Martin, & Fairbanks, 1997).*

they will have difficulty retrieving information (see Gagnon & Wagner, 2016, for review). Think of a time when you were beyond stressed and how this negatively affected your ability to retrieve a name or other piece of information that you could easily retrieve when the situation was calmer. If your client with SM is distracted with anxiety, they will likely have trouble focusing on the task at hand, holding information in their working memory, and/or retrieving information from their working memory. Also, if riddled with anxiety, they may be given many cues to self-monitor their communication responses but feel unable to do anything about their response. The result will be that despite cueing, they may, for example, fail to use a fluency strategy or may avoid communication due to extreme fear. Their pattern of little to no communication in certain environments may be so ingrained that they are not always aware of when they could be using fluency strategies. For example, you may be working with a school-aged client who stutters, and they have gained more comfort in talking with peers in class. As a next step, you and your client role-play talking with peers while beginning utterances with the fluency strategy of preparatory set. The client seems ready for this step. However, when you and the client are in the actual situation for the first time, their anxiety takes over. They are able to get out the practiced words, but do not use the practiced fluency strategy. They likely had every intention of using the strategy, but when they got into the new situation and their anxiety took over, they went right back to their original response. They may not even have been aware they didn't use the strategy.

Although no direct link has been found between cognitive flexibility and SM, links have been established between dysfunction of the prefrontal cortex (implicated in flexibility of behavior), cognitive flexibility, and anxiety (Lee & Orsillo, 2014; Park & Moghaddam, 2017). The research is still in early stages and as of now does not implicate differences in brain regions except when anxiety is provoked. Those with SM do not have difficulty with cognitive flexibility or problem solving in general. They have the skills to think of multiple causes to problem situations and multiple solutions to these situations. However, when placed in a fear-based situation, it may seem that they resort to only one response pattern: escape or avoidance. They may have what is known as "safety behaviors" they routinely do to maintain comfort, whether this be a secondary behavior or avoiding talking with certain speakers or in certain situations (Hofmann, 2007). This inflexibility is because the client has built strategies around what they know they can control. The things they feel they can control will give them more comfort in a situation. Are they being inflexible? Perhaps yes. But do they have a core problem with inflexibility? No. Again, it is rooted in anxiety. This is where we step in. By structuring the communication approach hierarchy to just the right amount of difficulty, we can help our clients control their anxiety to a level where they can use communication skills (including fluency strategies). Often before we have ever met our clients with SM, they likely have figured out some strategies to assist with communication, such as nonverbal options. We can help them to gradually build these nonverbal responses into more and more appropriate verbal interactions.

In a recent study comparing the joint attention skills of early school-aged children with mixed anxiety to those with SM and controls, those with SM demonstrated significantly less joint attention with their parents than the other two groups. The researchers concluded that the children with SM do not engage with their parents during stressful situations and therefore may not learn coping strategies for social situations (Nowakowski et al., 2011). This has the potential to have a negative impact upon a child's ability to self-regulate their behavior. Given these initial findings, the clinician should keep in mind that difficulties with self-regulation may result in increased difficulty for self-monitoring use of fluency strategies, regardless of what type of disfluency the strategies are designed for.

# MANAGEMENT STRATEGIES

Your first step in treatment of SM will be a language evaluation to rule out any co-occurring language disorder. A co-occurring language delay or disorder is not uncommon in SM (Hua & Major, 2016; McInnes et al., 2004). By definition, if a language disorder is considered to be the key reason a client is not speaking, then the diagnosis is not SM. However, a language delay or disorder should look the same in all situations, whereas SM will not. As previously noted, it may be best to begin with receptive language tests. Attempting an expressive language test may not ensure valid results. Even if your client does use some language in your room, in general, you run the risk of having trouble differentiating expressive language disorder from SM symptoms. It may be best to get an idea of receptive language level (perhaps starting with a receptive vocabulary test) and test expressive language later on in treatment, as the client becomes more verbal.

If receptive deficits are identified, they can be treated in the traditional manner. In terms of attempting to increase your client's time talking, you will build and work through a speaking hierarchy with your client. You will begin where you client is currently functioning. For example, if they are only exhibiting nonverbal communication in your office, they will only be required to use nonverbal communication for the first several sessions. Your client's speech may quickly progress beyond the nonverbal level in your treatment room. However, you will not expect or require it, thereby keeping the pressure low. For your first session, you may play a game that doesn't require much verbal response (perhaps a card or board game). Your client will be expected to do something nonverbal on their turn that communicates, "It's my turn." Perhaps they will blow a whistle, clap, or raise their hand. The idea is to make it fun with little pressure. When you take your turn, you will use the same nonverbal communication but pair it with the verbal, "My turn." By making that verbalization, you are modeling for the client what the next level of response should look like without requiring it. If the client is ready, you can have them use the same nonverbal communication the next week paired with the verbal, "My turn." If they are not quite ready, you continue to model the next level and try again for increased verbal the following week. Keeping activities and expectations consistent and routine is extremely important in decreasing anxiety. Anxiety is often triggered by the unknown (Walters & Charles, 1997): If I talk, how will the kids respond? How about my teacher? The more a client can learn exactly what to expect in your sessions, the more comfortable they will be. Once your client is able to produce a certain level of response on the hierarchy, you continue to make the verbal response longer and more complex. For example, you may move from a whistle blow (nonverbal response) to "My turn" to "It's my turn" to "I rolled a five" to "I rolled a five and I am going to move right here," etc. At each level, you need to determine when the time is right for the client to advance. You can use the feedback form at the end of this chapter to gain feedback on whether you are choosing a correct level for them to practice or whether you are choosing a level that is too scary. If the situation you are proposing makes your client feel in the "scared" range, then the task is too difficult, either in general or at that given time. If the client selects that the proposed situation makes them feel "happy," it may not be challenging enough for them. If the client selects that it makes them feel "okay," then this can be taken as the most appropriate level of challenge (i.e., not too easy or too scary).

Once the client advances to a conversational level in your room, you need to slowly build on what is expected in terms of communication with others. For example, perhaps you invite a peer into the room and the client and peer play a game. Or you work in the classroom, having the client speak with the teacher when no one else is in the room. Remember that even if the client does well in your room, when you add new components to the situation in your room (such as a peer) or try to take the skills outside of the room, your client may exhibit a regression. They may need to start back with nonverbal communication (while you model the nonverbal plus next level verbal, as in the beginning) and work their way through the hierarchy again. Realize that this is okay and the best way for

*Remember that even if the client does well in your room, when you add new components to the situation in your room (such as a peer) or try to take the skills outside of the room, your client may exhibit a regression.*

your client to become the most comfortable in all situations. They will need a lot of time and space for improvement. If they are pushed too far too soon, this could cause a larger regression (Dow, Sonies, Scheib, Moss, & Leonard, 1995). Always be mindful and aware that it is appropriate to move in "baby steps" according to your client's comfort level.

As you work with a client with SM, keep in mind that anxiety will be variable not only with the situation, but with the day in general. We all have days when our system is more taxed than others. Overall performance may be negatively affected on these days. If you've ever tried to change a response pattern of your own, you know that on certain days it seems easier to make progress than others. Using the guide at the end of this chapter can help you determine how far you can push a client on a given day. Whenever you talk with a client about approaching a given speaking situation and what is expected, you will need to assess how they feel about this situation. It is important to train others (parents and professionals) working with the client to assess the client's feelings before each activity and to understand that the client's response may change from day to day. Because those with SM may talk to us less than other clients, we need to find other ways of understanding their thoughts to help us design intervention that hits upon just the right challenge.

# WHEN TO WORK ON FLUENCY DISORDERS

If your client is reluctant to speak due to SM, then you need to focus on speaking and not fluency. You need to tease out whether your client is not talking due to fear of stuttering, due solely to SM, or both. A thorough history can help here. If your client is reported to speak freely at home and openly stutter without negative reaction, this is a good sign that their decreased communication is unrelated to stuttering. However, before drawing this conclusion for certain, it is important to find out if your client has any history of negative peer reactions to stuttering. It is possible that due to negative reactions about stuttering, your client has negative associations with certain contexts, such as the classroom, which may foster anxiety and avoidance. Keep in mind that regardless of the source of the initial anxiety, the anxiety may not necessarily manifest itself in a straightforward manner over time. For example, I once had a client whose anxiety sourced back to her brother and a friend laughing at her when she stuttered while doing a reading in church. One might think that her communication avoidance would then be in situations involving peers. That was true

*As you work with a client with SM, keep in mind that anxiety will be variable not only with the situation, but with the day in general.*

of situations with her brother and his friends, who were older than she was. But in school the anxiety resulted in avoidance of communicating with adults and comfort with peers. She perceived that adults might judge her speech, and peers would not. Any insight the speech-language clinician can gain about communication fear is important, with the caveat that the manifestation of communication avoidance does not always follow a linear path.

Fluency strategies can be introduced when the client is more comfortable with verbal communication. This is a delicate balance and may sometimes put you in a catch-22 situation. Your client may not be comfortable speaking if they know they are going to stutter. Therefore, in your individual speech sessions, you may need to try some fluency strategies to get them started while working through the speaking situation hierarchy designed for SM. You may have your client use a preparatory set at the word

> *Fluency strategies can be introduced when the client is more comfortable with verbal communication.*

level to get started. If their stuttering is severe, you may want to use fluency-enhancing methods such as choral speaking to get them started with success and gradually shape to other fluency strategies such as continuous phonation. If there is fear related to stuttering, it is best to work concurrently on changing perspectives on stuttering (see activities for changing cognitive misperceptions at the end of this chapter). For much of this, the child can respond nonverbally when needed. They can draw or write new responses to reframe communication attitudes. You also may work on desensitizing activities such as voluntary stuttering in your sessions.

Cognitive behavioral therapy approaches are often used to work with children with SM (Lang et al., 2016). These approaches are being used more and more with clients with fluency disorders (Menzies, Onslow, Packman, & O'Brian, 2009). Using such approaches involves helping a client change cognitive misperceptions. For example, instead of a client thinking, "I always stutter when I say my name," they can think, "Sometimes when I say my name, I get stuck. Prep set usually helps me get through my name when this happens "or" It's okay if I stutter on my name, people still want to know what it is." There is a sample sheet at the end of this chapter that provides an example of changing cognitive perceptions. Such activities are frequently used in fluency therapy and can be beneficial to the client who has a fluency disorder and SM.

# MEDICATION

As mentioned, the best strategy is for a speech-language clinician to work closely with a psychologist, psychiatrist, or counselor who understands SM. This allows for the most comprehensive treatment to be applied. A mental health professional familiar with SM will be able to advise the client's family whether medication is warranted. The recommendation for medication tends to be applied more commonly to individuals with long-standing issues surrounding SM that are resistant to improvement with therapy alone (Manassis, Oerbeck, & Overgaard, 2016). There has been some documentation of improvement in SM cases when taking selective serotonin reuptake inhibitors and phenelzine (an antidepressant). However, there are questions over the methods followed in many of the studies that suggest these results. Additionally, more study is needed regarding adverse effects (Manassis et al., 2016). As each case is individual, the speech-language clinician should work closely with the mental health professional to understand what medications are being prescribed and why and the potential impact and/or side effects that might be expected in the context of speech-language activities.

# SPEAKING HIERARCHY

## Week 1

- Play a game with basic turn-taking and no speech required.
  - Child blows horn to indicate "My turn."
  - Clinician blows horn then models saying, "My turn."
- Carryover assignment (to classroom, etc.) may be nonverbal.

## Week 2

- Play a game with basic turn-taking and no speech required.
  - Child blows horn and says (if ready), "My turn."
  - Clinician blows horn then models saying, "My turn. I rolled a five."
- Carryover assignment may require single-word responses with fluency strategies (if appropriate).

## Week 3

- Play a game with basic turn-taking and no speech required.
  - Child blows horn and says (if ready), "My turn. I rolled a five."
  - Clinician blows horn then models saying, "My turn. I rolled a five. I land here."
- Carryover assignment may require short-phrase responses with fluency strategies (if appropriate).

## Week 4

- Play a game with basic turn-taking and no speech required.
  - Child blows horn and says (if ready), "My turn. I rolled a five. I land here."
  - Clinician blows horn then models saying, "My turn. I rolled a five. I land here. I think I am going to win."
- Carryover assignment may require sentence-level responses with fluency strategies (if appropriate).

**Note**: Because most clients with SM will not be challenged by a home assignment, the clinician will need to work closely with the parent and/or teacher to design challenging yet achievable tasks (e.g., a short phrase or wave at a family outing, using a nonverbal signal to greet a teacher, etc.). Above all else, the clinician should make sure the client is comfortable with whatever the home or in-class assignment is.

# ACTIVITY 10-1:
## JUST THE RIGHT CHALLENGE CHECKLIST

I am going to try  _____

Talking about trying this out makes me feel:

☐  Happy ☺

☐  Okay ☺

☐  Scared ☹

# Activity 10-2:
## Stepping Stones to More Communication (Sample Hierarchy, Including Fluency Strategies):

1. Nonverbal response to signal your turn while playing a game (blowing a whistle, raising a hand, pointing to a card that says "my turn").

2. Pair nonverbal response with verbal "my turn."

3. Repeat previous step, adding preparatory set on "myyy turn."

4. Say "my turn" and add a sentence relevant to the game, for example, "I rolled a six."

5. Repeat previous step, adding preparatory set on "myyy turn" and "III rolled a six."

6. Answer an easy question before each turn (e.g., "Tell me how old you are").

7. Repeat previous step, adding preparatory set on sentence client says (e.g., "IIII am ten years old").

8. Ask each other simple closed-ended questions (that can be answered in a sentence) before each turn.

9. Repeat previous step, using preparatory set when asking and answering each questions.

10. Answer open-ended questions before each turn.

11. Repeat previous step, using preparatory set on first word of each sentence when answering open-ended questions.

**Notes:**
- The term *preparatory set* can be substituted with any relevant fluency strategies, such as emphasizing ending sounds, pausing, continuous phonation, etc.
- Hierarchy may vary depending upon client needs and comfort.
- In the current session, clinician should always model one step higher that client will be expected to do during the next session.

# ACTIVITY 10-3:
# PAUSING IS HARD WHEN I'M SCARED! PRACTICE FOR PAUSING (ATYPICAL FLUENCY, CLUTTERING)

It is hard to use pausing when I am scared to talk. When I am scared, I just want to get my words out quickly so they will be over with. I can practice using long pauses with my speech teacher. If I practice them where I am comfortable and use eye contact, it will be easier with other people. Also, in speech sessions, I will make the pauses extra-long so I get comfortable with these. But in real situations, when I am nervous, my pauses will be shorter. I have to practice longer so that I don't end up shortening them to nothing in real situations!

I can use pausing when:

- Reading

- Answering short questions

- Having a conversation

# ACTIVITY 10-4:
# IT'S HARD TO SAY SOMETHING QUICKLY:
# TIPS FOR USING PREPARATORY SET

The card game "War" can help teach clients how to use a fluency strategy in a fast-paced situation. Practicing this in a situation that's comfortable for the child is a great place to start.

*Materials:* A deck of playing cards

*Directions:* Client and clinician each put a card out and the player with the highest card takes all of the cards. The object of the game is to collect all the cards.

Incorporating the fluency strategy: Client and clinician practice preparatory set while placing down cards:

Client: IIIIII am putting down an ace

Clinician: IIIII am putting down a 2

Client: IIIII win the card

Through a Speed Round, clients can learn a way to insert themselves into a conversation with friends when it is fast paced and everyone is talking quickly by practicing a strategy proactively and quickly.

Client: IIIII have a 2

Clinician: IIIII have an ace

Client (says it first): IIII steal your card

If clinician was first to say "IIII win the card," they would get the card. But if the client is first to use the strategy, they get to steal the card, even though their card is the lower number. See also Activity 8-3.

# ACTIVITY 10-5:
# TALKING SOMETIMES MAKES ME FEEL BAD:
# CHANGING MY THOUGHTS

**Change your thoughts that have "always" or "never" in them to something really true**. For example, "I always stutter on every word." Is this really true? A more accurate statement might be, "I sometimes stutter when I talk. I can use strategies if I want to or I can just say what I want to say, even if I stutter."

**Change your thoughts that blame someone or something for your trouble talking**. For example, "It's my fault I stutter." Is this really true? Do you do it on purpose? A more accurate statement might be, "Stuttering is no one's fault; it just happens to some people when they talk. I am working on doing my best to manage it so that I feel in control of my speech."

**Change your thoughts about what happened one time**. For example, "I stuttered when I answered a question in class last week, so I will not raise my hand anymore because I will stutter." Do you know this is true? Have you tested it out? A more accurate statement might be, "Sometimes I stutter when I raise my hand. Whether I stutter or use my strategies on the answer, the teacher still wants to hear what I have to say."

When you change your thoughts about talking to things that are more true, it will make talking less scary for you. In the space below, write or draw some thoughts you have and how you might change them to be more true.

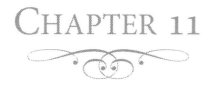

# CHAPTER 11

# GIFTED AND TALENTED

## WHO IS GIFTED?

The answer to this question may be different depending on the source. If one were to consider the multiple intelligences proposed by Howard Gardner (1983), then we are all gifted in different areas. Any readers who are parents or friends of parents have heard stories where children who are expected to be admitted to gifted and talented programs are rejected due to results of testing, teacher recommendations, and/or other requirements, which vary by school. Giftedness therefore seems difficult to define. It is important to note that giftedness used to be considered only in terms of intelligence quotient (IQ) score, and only recently has the "talented" portion of the "gifted and talented" label emerged. Talent is viewed in areas outside of traditional academic achievement. Most of the existing research focuses on children who are gifted in an academic sense rather than talented in other ways (Webb, 1993). For the purposes of this book, when I refer to gifted, I am referring to those who have been identified to fit within this category by their school in an academic rather than a talented sense. This is not to devalue talent, but rather to focus on proposed relations I will describe between cognitive and language skills and fluency.

The federal definition of giftedness in the United States is as follows:

> Students, children, or youth who give evidence of high achievement capability in areas such as intellectual, creative, artistic, or leadership capacity, or in specific academic fields, and who need services and activities not ordinarily provided by the school in order to fully develop those capabilities. (Elementary and Secondary Education Act of 1965)

Each state within the United States defines gifted and talented based upon this federal definition, but is not required to follow the exact federal definition (National Association for Gifted Children, 2017). Therefore, how gifted students are identified and defined varies by state. Some school districts use scores on ability and/or achievement tests. Whereas most clients we see are likely to have been identified within their school, other individuals may have been identified by testing outside of their school system. If a client has not been officially identified as gifted and/or talented, it is not within the scope

Scaler Scott, K.
*Fluency Plus: Managing Fluency Disorders in*
*Individuals With Multiple Diagnoses (pp 175-186).*
© 2018 Taylor & Francis Group.

of the speech-language clinician's practice to make this diagnosis, even if achievement and/or ability scores are known (through reports of cognitive testing) and traits presented by the client are judged to be in line with those who fit into the gifted category. However, understanding the traits of clients who present with gifted characteristics (described throughout this chapter), whether officially identified or not, may assist with more effective management of fluency disorders in this population.

## WHAT FLUENCY DISORDERS ARE COMMONLY FOUND IN THIS POPULATION?

There is currently no research supporting a link between fluency disorders and giftedness. Given that giftedness often represents above-average skills in specific areas, an uneven profile of development is possible. Uneven profiles of development have been identified in some populations of children with fluency disorders. There have been consistent findings in the literature regarding a link between early development of stuttering and language skills that are identified as weak in experimental tasks but not in standardized testing (Bloodstein & Bernstein Ratner, 2008). More recent testing suggests potential deficits in syntactic processing on event-related brain potentials among 6- to 7-year-old children who persisted in stuttering as compared to those who recovered from stuttering (Usler & Weber-Fox, 2015). An uneven profile of speech-language development is supported in preschool children who stutter (Anderson, Pellowski, & Conture, 2005), a small sample of children who clutter (Kidron, Scaler Scott, & Lozier, 2012), and a small sample of children with atypical disfluencies (Sutkowski, Tokach, Scaler Scott, 2015). It is important to note that an uneven profile of skills is not diagnostic criteria for giftedness, but may be present in both the gifted population and in some clients with fluency disorder. The speech-language clinician working with clients with disfluency should be cognizant of the characteristic features of giftedness and/or a client's identification as gifted and/or talented.

*...how gifted students are identified and defined varies by state.*

## MYTHS AND FACTS REGARDING THIS POPULATION

Many of the concerns regarding the social and/or emotional struggles encountered by those identified as gifted and/or talented are related to myths regarding how best to engage someone within this population. First, knowing that a child has high intellectual capability, a parent and/or teacher may have unrealistic expectations for that child's performance. This may fall into a number of areas. For example, it is often difficult for adults to remember that just because a child is superior to their chronological age cognitively, emotionally they may not be superior. It may be difficult for others to remember that a 7-year-old should only be expected to meet the emotional milestones of 7-year-old peers, even if their intellectual ability is superior to other 7-year-old peers (Roedell, 1984).

*...understanding the traits of clients who present with gifted characteristics, whether officially identified or not, may assist with more effective management of fluency disorders in this population.*

Another myth that may result in unrealistic expectations is that a gifted child will enjoy cognitive challenges of all kinds. Because things often come easily and quickly to gifted children, they are not always apt to put in extra work to complete more challenging tasks. Additionally, they may become frustrated when asked to do so, much to the surprise of adults around them (Roedell, 1984; Webb, 1993). Likewise, those who are gifted may be underachieving in school for a number of reasons. First, they may avoid more challenging tasks out of anxiety of failure. Second, they may underachieve to better fit in with same-age peers. Additionally, as giftedness is defined by variable criteria, it is important to understand that gifted children do not often excel in all areas. Therefore, for a client who is primarily gifted in mathematics, a challenging language arts task that is above their age level is not appropriate. It is very important for clinicians and parents to fully understand the criteria that were used to determine a gifted diagnosis in the child. In this way, realistic expectations for performance can be set (National Association for Gifted Children, 2017).

*...those who are gifted may be underachieving in school for a number of reasons.*

Another myth is that gifted children always have social difficulty. Those who are gifted may be more prone to social difficulties, but it is important to understand where these social difficulties originate. First, it may be that a child who is gifted has a difficult time relating socially to same-age peers with interests different from their own. Some who fit into the gifted population can also be focused on moral justice, which results in their attempting to enforce rules in a way that their same-age peers may not appreciate (Webb, 1993). Clients who are gifted often have high expectations of themselves and therefore may place these unrealistic expectations upon peers (Webb, 1993). Although debates remain for all findings, there is literature to support that those who fit into the category of "talented" are more likely to encounter social difficulties than those who fit into the category of "gifted." Another hypothesis is that a subset of those in the gifted and talented population have difficulties with social issues (Webb, 1993).

# EXECUTIVE FUNCTIONING ISSUES TO EXPECT IN THE GIFTED POPULATION

Attention issues have been found in the gifted population. Difficulties with attention to task have been hypothesized to be due to the fact that those who are gifted have trouble attending to tasks that are not challenging enough. Looking at another aspect of attention, because those who are gifted may be able to concentrate for long periods, they may have difficulty shifting attention once engaged and intensely focusing on a task (Webb, 1993). Another issue with attention may come out of the fact that those who are gifted may set high standards for themselves and put off tasks at which they feel they will fail. Therefore, although attention difficulties may be identified in a client who is gifted, the issues at their core may be more related to issues with perfectionism and/or frustration and boredom with inappropriate curriculum than true attention deficit disorders (Webb, 1993).

*...although attention difficulties may be identified in a client who is gifted, the issues at their core may be more related to issues with perfectionism and/or frustration and boredom with inappropriate curriculum than true attention deficit disorders (Webb, 1993).*

Because those who are gifted may avoid tasks that do not come easily to them, difficulties can be found in the area of task persistence. Gifted children often present with strengths in the area of memory (Hettinger Steiner & Carr, 2003). Given the fact that those who are gifted may have perfectionistic tendencies, they may set unrealistic goals for themselves (Webb, 1993). The client who is gifted may show strength in the area of problem solving (Hettinger Steiner & Carr, 2003). However, given moralistic views of rule systems (Webb, 1993), difficulties may be seen in the area of cognitive flexibility.

There is a subset of those in the gifted and talented population who are also diagnosed with other disabilities, such as attention deficit hyperactivity disorder (ADHD) or dyslexia. This subset is often not identified until later school years because their strong academic ability allows them to compensate

> *Because those who are gifted may avoid tasks that do not come easily to them, difficulties can be found in the area of task persistence.*

for relative weaknesses. Given the fact that there may be a concomitant diagnosis, the executive functioning deficits commonly associated with these diagnoses are possible. For example, it is possible for a child who is gifted and who has ADHD to be dealing with issues in the areas of working memory and response inhibition. The reader is referred to the chapters that correspond with relevant concomitant diagnoses when working with a gifted client who also has been diagnosed with one of these concomitant disorder categories.

# MANAGEMENT STRATEGIES

All management strategies will be based upon the findings regarding the characteristic traits of clients within the gifted population. The first of these strategies applies to when a gifted client needs to be scheduled in the context of a group session. Roedell (1984) makes an important analogy about grouping gifted students with students of average cognitive ability. The author explains that doing so equates to the same as placing a regular education student in a class for special education students. Because clients who are gifted may have more in common with older peers, the clinician may want to consider grouping by interest or cognitive level rather than by age. That being said, the clinician will also have to take into account the client's emotional level compared to older peers. The client may be a better fit with older peers cognitively, but not emotionally. This is something that needs further study. The clinician

> *The clinician is urged to consider the cognitive, social, and emotional dynamic of each group she or he is planning. The clinician should also consider the dynamics and values of the population from which each group is coming.*

is urged to consider the cognitive, social, and emotional dynamic of each group she or he is planning. The clinician should also consider the dynamics and values of the population from which each group is coming. For example, whereas some who are gifted come from a family where there is significant pressure to continue to do well academically, others may come from a family where academic ability is not valued and may even be ridiculed. Even if the clinician sets ground rules for these groupings, the grouping itself may lead to underachievement by the child who is gifted and talented. There is evidence that within certain cultures (Roedell, 1984), students are discouraged from seeking gifted and talented classifications, as they are seen not to fit in within their mainstream culture. Also, keep in mind that those who are gifted may ask questions at a level others do not, as they are believed to think more deeply and broadly (Webb, 1993) than their peers. This is another reason that when planning the therapy schedule, the right groupings are so important. Additionally, gifted students are more prone to isolation and depression (Dai, Moon, & Feldhusen, 1998). Therefore, group treatment with the right matches may prove to support a client's need to interact with others. As is true when working with any client with fluency disorders, it is best to keep open dialogue about healthy communication.

Given that a gifted client may exhibit perfectionistic tendencies and consequently decreased task persistence, the clinician may need to assist with realistic goal setting. The clinician can help the client set goals that are achievable within a relatively short period. Setting this up should help to maintain the client's focus. Reminding of previous successes will also be helpful. An example of an activity assisting with goal setting is included at the end of this chapter. An activity for helping a client to problem-solve frustrating situations is also included.

It has been found that those who are gifted rely on their superior cognitive skills rather than strategies, as their superior skills release them of the need for strategies (Hettinger Steiner & Carr, 2003). Therefore, the clinician may at times find it difficult to get a gifted client to "buy in" to strategy use. At times what I have found helpful is for clients with excessive non–stuttering-like disfluencies, cluttering, and/or atypical disfluencies to think about not what can make their talking easier, but what can make their talking be more easily understood by the listener. This sometimes results in a paradigm shift that allows the client to better buy in to strategy use. (See the end of the chapter for an activity focusing on this.) We must be careful to note that we are not telling a client who stutters, has healthy attitudes toward communicating, and chooses to openly stutter to use strategies for the benefit of their listener. Whether gifted or not, the choice to use stuttering strategies is an individual one. Making decisions about strategy use should be an ongoing dialogue between the speech-language clinician, clients, and families. The shift in thought about ease for the listener more applies to cases where the listener truly cannot follow the speaker's message, such as in cluttering, atypical disfluency (depending upon its presentation), and excessive non–stuttering-like disfluencies.

*Given that a gifted client may exhibit perfectionistic tendencies and consequently decreased task persistence, the clinician may need to assist with realistic goal setting.*

There is some controversy in the literature about differences in language development and its relationship to stuttering (see Bloodstein & Bernstein Ratner, 2008, for review). Recent studies have begun to investigate the interaction between language development in preschool children, external demands for the complexity of utterances produced, and emotional demands (such as whom a person is speaking with; see Hollister, Van Horne, & Zebrowski, 2016, for review). In investigating the relationship between internal language development and external demands for utterance length and complexity, Hollister et al. (2016) did find a relationship between decrease in disfluency among preschoolers who recovered from stuttering and increased grammatical skills. The authors concluded that as the gap between language ability and demand lessened, differences in children's disfluency could no longer be predicted by external factors such as utterance length and/or complexity. Thus, stronger internal language skills were hypothesized to contribute in a positive way to recovery from disfluency. Initial comparison of a sample of children with word-final disfluencies (WFDs) showed this same trend of decreased WFDs in children when the gap between skills and the demand of the situation was lessened. If a fluency client presents with scores on language testing that are relatively low compared to other skills but still within normal limits, it will be up to the clinician's discretion whether or not to address the relatively weak skills. The decision made will depend on the policies of the clinician's work setting and the client's family priorities. Trying to close the gap between areas to help even out a cognitive profile has assisted a small group of children with atypical disfluencies in decreasing the atypical disfluencies. Specifically, addressing and teaching compensatory strategies

*It has been found that those who are gifted rely on their superior cognitive skills rather than strategies, as their superior skills release them of the need for strategies (Hettinger Steiner & Carr, 2003).*

for language organization and working memory have resulted in decreased atypical disfluencies (Scaler Scott et al., 2013; Scaler Scott, Reeves, Block, Kidron, & Lozier, 2011). Caveats do apply as the improvements are correlated with the treatments rather than proven to be caused by the treatments. There is currently no research that has studied the impact of "evening out" (through compensatory strategy use or therapy targeting specific weak areas) a client's cognitive

*Making decisions about strategy use should be an ongoing dialogue between the speech-language clinician, clients, and families.*

profile on stuttering-like disfluencies. That being said, often clinicians working with preschoolers who stutter may turn to an indirect therapy program, where the client's caregivers increase pausing in their speech and place fewer speaking demands (i.e., rapid fire questions or asking for "performance speech" such as demonstrating what the child can say to relatives or family friends). The thought behind these modifications is that they help a client's system stay more balanced rather than taxed in particular areas (Starkweather, 1987). Some treatment studies have identified this program to work equally well as direct intervention programs (Sonneville-Koedoot, Stolk, Rietveld, & Franken, 2015; Yaruss, Coleman, & Hammer, 2006). See Chapter 5 for examples of indirect strategies. A case study of using an evening-out-of-profiles approach to atypical disfluency is presented at the end of this chapter.

Due to difficulties in shifting focus, when a gifted client is participating in a therapy activity such as a game, they may have such focus on game play that they have difficulty splitting their attention between playing the game and practicing strategies. I have found that talking with students about putting their full focus first on their practice and then on their turn in the game results in faster progress (as they are not dividing attention between focus on speech strategy and focus on game strategy) and helps to shift their thinking so that strategy practice can be more productive. Over time, clients can be taught to incorporate strategies in the context of taking their turn, but they may need more time initially to get to this level. See the activity at the end of this chapter focusing on splitting attention during strategy practice.

# CASE STUDY

Larry came to our clinic due to his mom's concerns regarding WFDs. Larry was 5 years, 11 months when his mother first sought treatment. She was referred by her current speech-language clinician, who had been treating Larry for language delay since the age 2. The clinician remarked that Larry had made significant gains in language in her years seeing him. In addition to the private speech-language treatment Larry was receiving, he underwent two child study team evaluations through his school district. After the initial testing, Larry was placed in a communication handicapped program and provided with extra help. He made significant gains in this program and through speech-language therapy. After his child study team re-evaluation, Larry was dismissed from services at his school. He continued to attend a private kindergarten classroom and to receive private speech-language services to address remaining articulation delays. At age 4, Larry began to exhibit typical stuttering characterized by part-word repetitions, prolongations, and blocks accompanied by physical tension. The clinician instructed the parents to use indirect strategies (i.e., increase pausing in speech, use modified questions). The clinician also began to teach the client direct strategies for disfluency, including rainbow speech, to which the clinician reported the client responded well. Over time, Larry's mother noticed a decrease in disfluency at the beginning of words and an increase in WFDs. Larry was bilingual, with his parents exclusively speaking French in the home and English outside the home. It was at the time that the WFDs developed that the clinician referred the client to me so that I could advise. The clinician had not heard the WFDs in any contexts in English, including spontaneous speech.

In reviewing Larry's records, he presented with a profile characterized by a general IQ score that was judged to be within normal limits. However, because of gaps in the score, the overall score was judged to not be an accurate representation of Larry's skills. Larry presented with superior visuospatial skills (evidence of high achievement in this area) and slightly below-average language skills. I began testing Larry in various areas of language and memory. He did not present with any WFDs during the first two testing sessions, where tasks completed included structured standardized testing (such as picture naming) and conversational speech. His mother brought in a video showing Larry using WFDs in French while explaining things to his family. Larry's mom indicated this speech context of explaining was the context that brought about the disfluencies in French. On the final day of testing, Larry was asked to retell stories about books he had read while looking at pictures of each story. It was during this context that the first WFDs in English were seen. In both English and French, increased formulation demands seemed to result in WFDs.

The following table lists Larry's scores. We spoke with his clinician about closing the gaps in the specific language areas of organization and grammar. Although specific standardized scores did not suggest difficulties with grammar or organization, qualitative signs were noted during testing, including frustration when attempting to retrieve words and/or ideas, and some immature grammatical forms in conversational speech. Grammatical skills were not considered to be behind given the fact that this client was developing two languages, which often results in what looks on the surface to be a delay before both languages "catch up" (Paul & Norbury, 2012). However, working with the hypothesis that the stress on his system related to these relative weaknesses may have correlated with disfluencies, I instructed the clinician to work on strengthening these areas. We also had her focus on using exercises to potentially strengthen his working memory, an area of weakness in testing. Over time, Larry's WFDs dissipated.

| TEST | NORMS | CLIENT 5-9; 5-10 |
|---|---|---|
| Peabody Picture Vocabulary Test 4 (PPVT-4) | Standard Score: 100 + or − 15<br>Percentile Rank: 50 + or − 25<br>Raw Score English: 89<br>Raw Score French: 99 | Standard Score English: 97<br>Percentile Rank English: 42<br>Standard Score French: 104<br>Percentile Rank French: 61<br>CA: 5-9 |
| Expressive Vocabulary Test 2 (EVT-2) | Standard Score: 100 + or − 15<br>Percentile Rank: 50 + or − 25<br>Raw Score English: 71<br>Raw Score French: 76 | Standard Score English: 97<br>Percentile Rank English: 42<br>Standard Score French: 101<br>Percentile Rank French: 53<br>CA: 5-10 |
| Test of Auditory Processing Skills (TAPS-3):<br>Word Memory | Scaled Score: 10 + or − 3<br>Percentile Rank: 50 = or − 25<br>Raw Score: 5 | Scaled Score: 3<br>Percentile Rank: 1<br>CA: 5-9 |
| Test of Auditory Processing Skills (TAPS-3):<br>Sentence Memory | Scaled Score: 10 + or − 3<br>Percentile Rank: 50 = or − 25<br>Raw Score: 6 | Scaled Score: 3<br>Percentile Rank: 1<br>CA: 5-9 |
| Comprehensive Test of Phonological Processing 2 (CTOPP-2):<br>Memory for Digits | Scaled Score: 10 + or − 3<br>Percentile Rank: 50 = or − 25<br>Raw Score: 12 | Scaled Score: 8<br>Percentile Rank: 25<br>CA: 5-10 |
| Comprehensive Test of Phonological Processing 2 (CTOPP-2):<br>Nonword Repetition | Scaled Score: 10 + or − 3<br>Percentile Rank: 50 = or − 25<br>Raw Score: 13 | Scaled Score: 9<br>Percentile Rank: 37<br>CA: 5-10 |
| Clinical Evaluation of Language Fundamentals (CELF-4):<br>Recalling Sentences | Scaled Score: 10 + or − 3<br>Percentile Rank: 50 = or − 25<br>Raw Score: 30 | Scaled Score: 9<br>Percentile Rank: 37<br>CA: 5-10 |
| Clinical Evaluation of Language Fundamentals (CELF-4):<br>Understanding Spoken Paragraphs | Scaled Score: 10 + or − 3<br>Percentile Rank: 50 = or − 25<br>Raw Score: 8 | Scaled Score: 9<br>Percentile Rank: 37<br>CA: 5-10 |
| Clinical Evaluation of Language Fundamentals (CELF-3):<br>Word Associations | Standard Score: 100 + or − 15<br>Percentile Rank: 50 + or − 25<br>Raw Score English: 19<br>Raw Score French: 10 | Scaled Score English: 8<br>Percentile Rank English: 25<br>Scaled Score French: 4<br>Percentile Rank French: 2 |

**Notes**: Two chronological ages are provided, as Larry was tested over a 3-day period and had his birthday during that period. Also, testing items for selected tests were administered in both language with the assistance of Larry's mother, who was bilingual French/English. Standard Scores represent an estimate only, as English norms were used in both cases.

# ACTIVITY 11-1: I THINK I NEED HELP! GUIDE TO IDENTIFYING FRUSTRATION AND DEVELOPING SELF-REGULATION

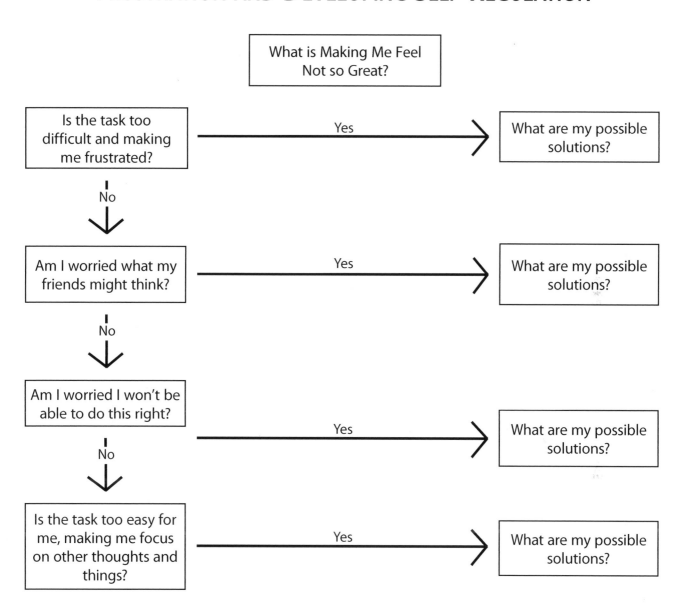

# ACTIVITY 11-2:
# THINGS I CAN DO TO HELP OTHERS FOLLOW MY MESSAGE: HELP WITH CLUTTERING, ATYPICAL DISFLUENCY, EXCESSIVE NON–STUTTERING-LIKE DISFLUENCIES

Things I can change about my speech to help the listener follow me:

• Put in pausing (so the listener has time to process the information).


• Give enough background information.


• When I use pronouns like "he," "she," or "it," make sure my listener knows who or what I am talking about.

**Directions**: Choose one of the three things from the list above to work on. Then tell your speech-language clinician a story. The story can be made up or something that really happened to you. Try to talk for about 5 minutes. While talking, raise your hand each time you focus on the skill that you have chosen. This will help your speech-language clinician know that you are actively monitoring this skill. Work with your speech-language clinician on developing a signal they can give you so that they can remind you of your goal as needed. Record how you did in the space below.

Goal I focused on:




How I did:




Goal I focused on:




How I did:

# ACTIVITY 11-3:
# SETTING REALISTIC GOALS

Everyone chooses goals to work on to improve something about themselves. There are smart ways for choosing a goal. **You should make sure that your goal is:**

- Not too easy (or you may get bored trying to work on it)

- Not too hard (or you may get frustrated trying to work on it)

**When you think about whether your goal is too hard or too easy, think about:**

- **Who** you are speaking with

- **Where** you are speaking

- **When** you are speaking

- **How** you are feeling

For all of these areas, you should choose what feels just right. For example, if you are working on using prep set and you have mastered it in the room having a conversation with your speech teacher, that level is too easy. But if you have a lot of trouble talking when you are at recess or feeling tired, then those times and places might be too hard. You might need to choose a situation in between, such as when talking to parents at home in a quiet room. Planning out what you will practice when with your speech teacher helps you make the best choices for you!

You also have to set a realistic number of times you will do this. Remember that realistic means you can complete this goal correctly that many times with little stress. It is important to not expect yourself to get it right every time the first time. No one usually can do this. If they can, it means the goal they picked is too easy for them! Once you pick a goal, try it out and see if you can get it right about 70% or 80% of the time. If you can, you've chosen the right thing to work on and should keep working on it until you get to 90% consistently and the goal is now too easy for you.

**Example goal:**
*I will use prep set for one question in each of my classes during a school day.*

# ACTIVITY 11-4:
# SHIFTING FOCUS

Choose a game to play with your speech-language clinician. Before you take a turn, put all your energy into practicing your speech goal. When you practice focusing only upon the goal and not upon the game or anything else going on in the room, this will help you put just the right amount of energy into practicing your goal. If you divide your energy between practicing the goal and thinking about the game (and maybe your next move), you will need twice as long to practice your goal, as you won't have your full attention on it. So put your full attention on the goal and work smarter and not harder. After you finish practicing your goal and it is your turn in the game, put your full attention on taking your turn and making your move!

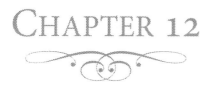

# CHAPTER 12

# CONCLUDING THOUGHTS

If you've made it this far in the book, I am hoping that you have gained the following:

- New information regarding what we know about the different types of fluency disorders: stuttering, cluttering, atypical disfluency, and excessive non–stuttering-like disfluency
- Strategies for differentiating fluency disorders and prioritizing whether a fluency disorder needs to be addressed clinically or merely monitored
- Increased awareness about what types of fluency disorders to expect in certain populations so that the possibility of these can be "on your radar" during assessment
- Awareness of the executive functioning deficits that might be encountered in fluency disorders and concomitant diagnoses, definitions of these deficits, and an understanding of how these deficits may play out in treatment
- Ideas for effectively determining the root cause of executive functioning deficits and strategies for managing these appropriately
- An understanding of concomitant disorders with which you were less familiar
- Practical ideas for combining fluency work with work on the communication goals of concomitant diagnoses
- Ideas about how to balance treatment priorities
- Ideas about how to determine when work in each concomitant area needs to be kept separate from fluency work and when two or more areas can be combined

This book attempted to cover commonly encountered concomitant diagnoses, but could not cover every diagnosis that might be concomitant to a fluency disorder. Hopefully you will take the principles outlined and apply them to understanding the characteristic features of any new populations you encounter. It seems as though the job of the speech-language clinician is becoming more and not less complex in terms of the diagnoses encountered. It is my hope that this book is just one of many you own that help you to deal with the complexity in a productive manner.

This book was meant to provide the reader with an overview of the different types of fluency disorders, research information about each disorder that may inform clinical practice, methods for

Scaler Scott, K.
*Fluency Plus: Managing Fluency Disorders in
Individuals With Multiple Diagnoses (pp 187-189).*
© 2018 Taylor & Francis Group.

differential diagnosis, the basics of treatment for each fluency disorder, and ideas and principles for treatment of fluency disorders with concomitant diagnoses. Entire volumes are written on the specifics of each concomitant diagnosis and each fluency diagnosis. Additionally, entire volumes are written on specific treatment techniques, such as working on

*While we are waiting for the evidence to arrive, we still have clients who have communication needs to treat.*

the affective and cognitive components of stuttering. I encourage the reader to refer to the references list at the end of this book and the Recommended Resources list that follows this chapter for more in-depth information regarding diagnoses.

I would like to impart to you some final thoughts about working with "fluency plus" disorders. I firmly believe that working in this manner and following these principles has helped me provide better care each day.

**Don't be afraid to ask questions**. I once had a supervisor who wrote in my work performance evaluation that she loved the way I "fearlessly asked questions." I have never considered myself to be fearless, and at the time I didn't think much about this comment. It has only been in recent years, when I sit on the other side of class participation as a college professor, that I have come to fully understand what she meant. For whatever reason, I was never the one in college whose hand was always up to ask a question. But when I began full-time clinical work, my mind was constantly (and still is) churning with questions: What's going on right now? How can I make the next session better? Are my colleagues seeing these behaviors too? I feel that the constant

*Understanding your limitations and referring to appropriate professionals are also necessary components of a complete plan of care.*

search for new information has served my clients well. It has helped me better understand their behaviors and their responses to treatment activities. It also has helped me avoid misjudging a behavior as communicating something it really is not (e.g., communicating "I need help" vs. "I don't want to pay attention right now"). Although there are general principles and patterns that we see in each concomitant disorder, each client, disorder, and situation will bring about more and more questions. Seeking out the answers to these questions is really necessary given the complexity of the cases we are presented with.

**Don't be afraid to acknowledge what you don't know (or the field doesn't know)**. The more disorder categories we treat, the more our knowledge base grows. However, we cannot know it all. Although there may be situations where administrators are short-sighted in understanding the limitations we may have (for example, maybe we see one fluency case per year in our given work setting), and the fact that the field of speech-language pathology has become quite specialized, it is our job to educate them about this. You should not be expected to do or know it all. Likewise, there are limitations to the research we have on different approaches. While we are waiting for the evidence to arrive, we still have clients who have communication needs to treat. I find that acknowledging with clients and families what is known and unknown in our field before beginning treatment is something that they truly understand and appreciate.

**Don't be afraid to collaborate and/or refer**. With the earlier comment about acknowledging your limitations, realize that "fluency plus" disorders often need a team approach. Collaborating with other professionals is always helpful in our field, but often necessary with "fluency plus" clients. Understanding your limitations and referring to appropriate professionals are also necessary components of a complete plan of care.

**Don't be afraid to go outside of your field for resources**. Having worked on teams with reading specialists, psychologists, neuropsychologists, occupational and physical therapists, art therapists, and classroom teachers, I have been exposed to many resources that are not specific to speech-language pathology. By delving into these resources, I have gained a broader perspective about all of the issues surrounding "fluency plus" clients. I can take the stance that these issues are not my area (and, of course, I would collaborate and/or refer to needs outside my area), but the fact is that the behaviors may present themselves in treatment whether they are my area or not. Therefore, it's been beneficial for me to understand them from multiple perspectives.

I thank you for embarking on this journey with me and for the work that you are doing and will do with your clients. Our clients live courageously each day managing the challenges their communication disorder(s) present. As the complexity of cases increase, we must rise to the challenge of living just as courageously and learning all we can to have a positive impact upon their communication success.

# Recommended Resources

Barkley, R. A. (2005). *ADHD and the nature of self-control*. New York, NY: The Guilford Press.

Cheasman, C., Everard, R., & Simpson, S. (Eds.). (2013). *Stammering Therapy from the Inside: New Perspectives on Working with Young People and Adults*. Surrey, England: J&R Publishing Services Ltd.

Chmela, K., & Reardon, N. (2001). *The School-aged Child Who Stutters: Working Effectively with Attitudes and Emotions*. Memphis, TN: Stuttering Foundation of America.

Hallowell, E. M., & Ratey, J. J. (1994). *Driven to distraction: Recognizing and coping with Attention Deficit Disorder from childhood through adulthood*. New York, NY: Pantheon.

Hodson, B., & Paden, E. (1983). *Targeting Intelligible Speech: A Phonological Approach to Remediation*. London, England: College Hill Press, Inc.

Kelman, E., & Nicholas, A. (2011). *Practical Intervention for Early Childhood Stammering: Palin PCI Approach (A Speechmark Practical Therapy Resource)*. London, England: Routledge.

Myers, F. L. (2011). Treatment of cluttering: A cognitive-behavioral approach centered on rate control. In D. Ward & K. Scaler Scott (Eds.), *Cluttering: Research, Intervention and Education*. East Sussex, England: Psychology Press.

Myers, F. L., & Bradley, C. L. (1992). Clinical management of cluttering from a synergistic framework. In F. L. Myers & K. O. St. Louis (Eds.), *Cluttering: A clinical perspective* (pp. 85–106). Leicester, England: FAR Communications.

Reardon-Reeves, N., & Yaruss, J.S. (2013). *School-aged Stuttering Therapy: A Practical Guide*. Stuttering Therapy Resources, Inc.

Scaler Scott, K. (2011). Cluttering and autism spectrum disorders. In D. Ward & K. Scaler Scott (Eds.), *Cluttering: Research, Intervention and Education*. East Sussex, England: Psychology Press.

Scaler Scott, K., & Ward, D. (2013). *Managing Cluttering: A Comprehensive Guidebook of Activities*. Austin, TX: Pro-Ed, Inc.

Scaler Scott, K., Ward, D. & St. Louis, K. O. (2010). Paul: Treatment of Cluttering in a School-aged Child. In S. Chabon and E. Cohn (Eds.), *The Communication Disorders Casebook: Learning by Example* (pp. 261–272). Boston, MA: Pearson.

Singer, B.D., Bashir, A.S. (1999). What are executive functions and self-regulations and what do they have to do with language-learning disorders? *Language, Speech, and Hearing Services in Schools, 30*(3), 265–273.

Yaruss, J.S., & Reardon-Reeves, N. (2017). *Early Childhood Stuttering Therapy: A Practical Guide*. Stuttering Therapy Resources, Inc.

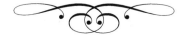

# REFERENCES

Agam, Y., Joseph, R. M., Barton, J. J., & Manoach, D. S. (2010). Reduced cognitive control of response inhibition by the anterior cingulate cortex in autism spectrum disorders. *Neuroimage, 52*(1), 336–347.

Ambrose, N. G., & Yairi, E. (1999). Normative disfluency data for early childhood stuttering. *Journal of Speech, Language, and Hearing Research, 42*(4), 895–909.

American Psychiatric Association. (1987). *Diagnostic and statistical manual of mental disorders* (3rd ed., Rev. ed.). Washington, DC: American Psychiatric Association.

American Psychiatric Association. (1987). *Diagnostic and statistical manual of mental disorders* (4th ed.). Washington, DC: American Psychiatric Association.

American Psychiatric Association. (2013). *Desk reference to the diagnostic criteria from DSM-5*. Washington, DC: American Psychiatric Association.

Anderson, J. D. & Conture, E. G. (2000). Language abilities of children who stutter: A preliminary study. *Journal of Fluency Disorders, 25*(4), 283–304.

Anderson, J. D., Pellowski, M. W., & Conture, E. G. (2005). Childhood stuttering and dissociations across linguistic domains. *Journal of Fluency Disorders, 30*, 219–253.

Anderson, J. D., & Wagovich, S. A. (2010). Relationships among linguistic processing speed, phonological working memory, and attention in children who stutter. *Journal of Fluency Disorders, 35*(3), 216–234.

Andreasen, N. C., & Grove, W. M. (1986). Thought, language, and communication in schizophrenia: Diagnosis and prognosis. *Schizophrenia Bulletin, 12*(3), 348–359.

Antrop, I., Stock, P., Verte, S., Wiersema, J. R., Baeyens, D., & Roeyers, H. (2006). ADHD and delay aversion: The influence of non-temporal stimulation on choice for delayed rewards. *Journal of Child Psychology and Psychiatry, 47*(11), 1152–1158.

Arndt, J., & Healey, E. C. (2001). Concomitant disorders in school-age children who stutter. *Language, Speech, and Hearing Services in Schools, 32*(2), 68–78.

Baddeley, A. (1996). Exploring the central executive. *The Quarterly Journal of Experimental Psychology: Section A, 49*(1), 5–28.

Bakker, K., Myers, F. L., Raphael, L. J., & St. Louis, K. O. (2011). A preliminary comparison of speech rate, self-evaluation, and disfluency of people who speak exceptionally fast, clutter, or speak normally. In D. Ward & K. Scaler Scott (Eds.), *Cluttering: Research, Intervention and Education*. East Sussex, England: Psychology Press.

Barkley, R. A. (1997). Behavioral inhibition, sustained attention, and executive functions: Constructing a unifying theory of ADHD. *Psychological Bulletin, 121*(1), 65–94.

Barkley, R. A. (2005). *ADHD and the nature of self-control*. New York, NY: The Guilford Press.

Bashir, A. S., Grahamjones, F., & Yale Bostwick, F. (1984). A touch-cue method of therapy for developmental verbal apraxia. *Seminars in Speech and Language, 5*(2), 127–137.

Belser R. C., & Sudhalter, V. (2001). Conversational characteristics of children with fragile X syndrome: Repetitive speech. *American Journal on Mental Retardation, 106*(1), 28–38.

Bernstein, N. E. (1981). Are there constraints on childhood disfluency? *Journal of Fluency Disorders, 6*(4), 341–350.

Bernstein Ratner, N. (1997). Stuttering: A psycholinguistic perspective. In R. Curlee & G. Siegel (Eds.), *Nature and treatment of stuttering: New directions* (2nd ed., pp. 99–127). Needham, MA: Allyn & Bacon.

Bernthal, J. E., Bankson, N. W., & Flipsen, P., Jr. (2012). *Articulation and phonological disorders: Speech sound disorders in children* (7th ed.). New York, NY: Allyn & Bacon.

Bichon [Digital image]. (n.d.). Retrieved from dooziedog.com.

Bichon Confused [Digital image]. (n.d.). Retrieved from dooziedog.com.

Blood, G. W., Blood, I. M., & Tellis, G. W. (1999). Attention and laterality preferences in children who clutter. *Acoustical Society of America, 106*, 2244.

Blood, G. W., Blood, I. M., & Tellis, G. W. (2000). Auditory processing and cluttering in young children. *Acoustical Society of America, 90*(2), 631–639.

Blood, G. W., Ridenour, V. J., Jr., Qualls, C. D., & Hammer, C. H. (2003). Co-occuring disorders in children who stutter. *Journal of Communication Disorders, 36*, 427–448.

Scaler Scott, K.
*Fluency Plus: Managing Fluency Disorders in Individuals With Multiple Diagnoses (pp 191-197).*
© 2018 Taylor & Francis Group.

Blood, I. M., Blood, G. W., & Tellis, G. W. (1997). Literacy differences between children who clutter and stutter. *Acoustical Society of America, 101,* 3126.

Bloodstein, O. (2002). Early stuttering as a type of language difficulty. *Journal of Fluency Disorders, 27,* 163–166.

Bloodstein, O. (2006). Some empirical observations about early stuttering: A possible link to language development. *Journal of Communication Disorders, 39,* 185–91.

Bloodstein, O., & Bernstein Ratner, N. (2008). *A handbook on stuttering* (6th ed.). Clifton Park, NY: Delmar.

Boscolo, B., Bernstein Ratner, N., & Rescorla, L. (2002). Fluency of school-aged children with a history of specific expressive language impairment: An exploratory study. *American Journal of Speech-Language Pathology, 11,* 41–49.

Boudreau, D., & Costanza-Smith, A. (2011). Assessment and treatment of working memory deficits in school-age children: The role of the speech-language pathologist. *Language, Speech, and Hearing Services in Schools, 42,* 152–166.

Braun, A. R., Varga M., Stager S., Schulz G., Selbie S., Maisog JM., . . . Ludlow C. L. (1997). Altered patterns of cerebral activity during speech language production in developmental stuttering: An H2(15)O positron emission tomography study. *Brain, 120,* 761–784.

Bretherton-Furness, J. *Phonological encoding in adults who clutter and adults who stutter* (Unpublished doctoral dissertation). University of Reading, Reading.

Bretherton-Furness, J., & Ward, D. (2012). Lexical access, story retelling, and sequencing skills in adults who clutter and those who do not. *Journal of Fluency Disorders, 37,* 214–224.

Brown, S., Ingham, R. J., Ingham, J. C., Laird, A. R., & Fox, P. T. (2005). Stuttered and fluent speech production: An ALE meta-analysis of functional neuroimaging studies. *Human Brain Mapping, 25,* 105–117.

Brundage, S. B., Whelan, C. J., & Burgess, C. M. (2013). Brief report: Treating stuttering in an adult with autism spectrum disorder. *Journal of Autism and Developmental Disorders, 43*(2)1–7.

Brutten, E. J., & Shoemaker, D. J. (1967). *The modification of stuttering.* Englewood Cliffs, NJ: Prentice-Hall.

Brutten, G. J., & Vanryckeghem, M. (2006). *Behavior assessment battery for school-age children who stutter.* San Diego, CA: Plural Publishing, Inc.

Byrd, C. T., Vallely, M., Anderson, J. D., & Sussman, H. (2012). Nonword repetition and phoneme elision in adults who do and do not stutter. *Journal of Fluency Disorders, 37*(3), 188–201.

Camarata, S. M. (1989). Final consonant repetition: A linguistic perspective. *Journal of Speech and Hearing Disorders, 52,* 174–178.

Chang, S. E., Erickson, K. I., Ambrose, N. G., Hasegawa-Johnson, M. A., & Ludlow, C. L. (2008). Brain anatomy differences in childhood stuttering. *Neuroimage, 39*(3): 1333–1344. doi:10.1016/j.neuroimage.2007.09.067

Chang, S. E., Kenney, M. K., Loucks, T. M. J., & Ludlow, C. L. (2009). Brain activation abnormalities during speech and non-speech in stuttering speakers. *Neuroimage, 46*(1), 201–212. doi:10/1016/j.neuroimage.2009.01.066

Chmela, K., & Reardon, N. (2001). *The school-age child who stutters: Working effectively with attitudes and emotions.* Memphis, TN: Stuttering Foundation of America.

Clark, H. H., & Fox Tree, J. E. (2002). Using uh and um in spontaneous speaking. *Cognition, 84,* 73–111.

Cohen, D., Pichard, N., Tordjman, S., Baumann, C., Burglen, L., Excoffier, E., Héron, D. (2005). Specific genetic disorders and autism: Clinical contribution towards their identification. *Journal of Autism and Developmental Disorders, 35,* 103–116. http://dx.doi.org/10.1007/s10803-004-1038-2

Colle, L., Baron-Cohen, S., Wheelwright, S., & van der Lely, H. J. K. (2008). Narrative discourse in adults with high-functioning autism or Asperger syndrome. *Journal of Autism Developmental Disorders, 38,* 28–40.

Constable, P. A., Ring, M., Bowler, D. M., & Gaigg, S. B. (2017). Problem solving styles in autism spectrum disorder and the development of higher cognitive functions. *Autism, 1,* 1362361317691044.

Conture, E. G. (2001). *Stuttering: Its nature, diagnosis, and treatment.* Needham Heights, MA: Allyn & Bacon.

Conture, E. G., Kelly, E. M., & Walden, T. A. (2013). Temperament, speech and language: An overview. *Journal of Communication Disorders, 46*(2), 125–142.

Cosyns, M., Mortier, G., Corthals, P., Janssens, S., & Van Borsel, J. (2010). Word-final prolongations in an adult male with neurofibromatosis type 1. *Journal of Fluency Disorders, 35*(3), 235–245. doi:10.1016/j.jfludis.2010.05.001

Cosyns, M., Mortier, G., Janssens, S., Saharan, N., Stevens, E., & Van Borsel, J. (2010). Speech fluency in neurofibromatosis type 1. *Journal of Fluency Disorders, 35*(1), 59–69. doi:10.1016/j.jfludis.2010.01.002

Dai, D. Y., Moon, S. M., & Feldhusen, J. F. (1998). Achievement motivation and gifted students: A social cognitive perspective. *Educational Psychologist, 33*(2–3), 45–63.

Daly, D. (1993). Cluttering: The Orphan of Speech-Language Pathology. *American Journal of Speech-Language Pathology, 2,* 6-8. doi:10.1044/1058-0360.0202.06

Daly, D. A., & Cantrell, R. P. (2006a, July). Cluttering inventory, experimental version (2003). *Cluttering: Characteristics identified as diagnostically significant by 60 fluency experts.* Presented at the Fifth World Congress on Fluency Disorders, Dublin.

Daly, D. A., & Cantrell, R. P. (2006b, July). Predictive cluttering inventory (2006). *Cluttering: Characteristics identified as diagnostically significant by 60 fluency experts.* Presented at the Fifth World Congress on Fluency Disorders, Dublin.

De Nil, L. F., Beal, D. S., Lafaille, S. J., Kroll, R. M., Crawley, A. P., & Gracco, V. L. (2008). The effects of simulated stuttering and prolonged speech on the neural activation patterns of stuttering and nonstuttering adults. *Brain and Language, 107*(2), 114–123.

De Nil, L. F., Kroll, R. M., Lafaille, S. J., & Houle, S. (2003). A positron emission tomography study of short- and long-term treatment effects on functional brain activation in adults who stutter. *Journal of Fluency Disorders, 28,* 357–380.

Dewey, J. (2005). My experiences with cluttering. Online conference at the Eighth Annual International Stuttering Awareness Day (ISAD).

Dodd, B., Holm, A., Crosbie, S., & McIntosh, B. (2006). A core vocabulary approach for management of inconsistent speech disorder. *Advances in Speech-Language Pathology, 8*(3), 220–230.

Doi M., Nakayasu H., Soda T., Shimoda K., Ito A., & Nakashima K. (2003). Brainstem infarction presenting with neurogenic stuttering. *Internal Medicine, 42*(9), 884–887.

Dow, S. P., Sonies, B. C., Scheib, D., Moss, S. E., & Leonard, H. L. (1995). Practical guidelines for the assessment and treatment of selective mutism. *Journal of the American Academy of Child & Adolescent Psychiatry, 34*(7), 836–846.

Dummit, E. S., Klein, R. G., Tancer, N. K., Asche, B., Martin, J., & Fairbanks, J. A. (1997). Systematic assessment of 50 children with selective mutism. *Journal of the American Academy of Child & Adolescent Psychiatry, 36*(5), 653–660.

Dunn, L. M. & Dunn, D. M. (2007). *Peabody Picture Vocabulary Test, Fourth Edition (PPVT-4).* San Antonio, TX: Pearson.

Dykens, E. M., Roof, E., & Hunt-Hawkins, H. (2017). Cognitive and adaptive advantages of growth hormone treatment in children with Prader-Willi syndrome. *Journal of Child Psychology and Psychiatry, 58*(1), 64–74.

Eggers, K., DeNil, L., & Van den Bergh, B. (2010). Temperamental dimensions of stuttering, voice disordered and typically developing children. *Journal of Fluency Disorders, 35,* 355–372.

Eichorn, N., Marton, K., Schwartz, R.G., Melara, R.D., & Pirutinsky, S. (2016). Does working memory enhance or interfere with speech fluency in adults who do and do not stutter? Evidence from a dual-talk paradigm. *Journal of Speech, Language, Hearing Research, 59,* 415–429.

Engelhardt, P. E., Corley, M., Nigg, J. T., & Ferreira, F. (2010). The role of inhibition in the production of disfluencies. *Memory & Cognition, 38*(5), 617–628.

Esteller, M. (2011). Non-coding RNAs in human disease. *Nature Reviews Genetics, 12,* 861–874. doi:10.1038/nrg3074

Fisher, B. L., Allen, R., & Kose, G. (1996). The relationship between anxiety and problem-solving skills in children with and without learning disabilities. *Journal of Learning Disabilities, 29*(4), 439–446. doi:10.1177/002221949602900412

Fox, P. T., Ingham, R. J., Ingham, J. C., Hirsch, T. B., Downs, J. H., Martin, C., . . . Lancaster, J. L. (1996). A PET study of the neural systems of stuttering. *Nature, 382,* 158–161.

Fox, P. T., Ingham, R. J., Ingham, J. C., Zamarripa, F., Xiong, J. H., & Lancaster, J. L. (2000). Brain correlates of stuttering and syllable production: A PET performance-correlation analysis. *Brain, 123*(10), 1985–2004.

Fratantoni, J. M., DeLaRosa, B. L., Didehbani, N., Hart, J. Jr., & Kraut, M. A. (2016). Electrophysiological correlates of word retrieval in traumatic brain injury. *Journal of Neurotrauma, 33,* 1–5.

Gagnon, S. A., & Wagner, A. D. (2016). Acute stress and episodic memory retrieval: Neurobiological mechanisms and behavioral consequences. *Annals of the New York Academy of Sciences, 1369*(1), 55–75.

Gardner, H. (1993). *Multiple intelligences.* New York, NY: Basic Books.

Garnett, E. O., & St. Louis, K. O. (2014). Verbal time estimation in cluttering. *Contemporary Issues in Communication Science and Disorders, 41,* 196–209.

German, D. J. (1992). Word-finding intervention for children and adolescents. *Topics in Language Disorders, 13*(1), 33–50.

German, D. J. (2015). *Test of Word Finding, Third Edition.* Austin, TX: PRO-ED, Inc.

Gertner, B. L., Rice, M. L., & Hadley, P. A. (1994). Influence of communicative competence on peer preferences in a preschool classroom. *Journal of Speech and Hearing Research, 37,* 913–923.

Gillam, R. B. & Pearson, N.A. (2017). *Test of Narrative Language, Second Edition (TNL-2).* Austin, TX: PRO-ED, Inc.

Goldman, R. & Fristoe, M. (2015). *Goldman-Fristoe Test of Articulation 3 (GFTA-3).* San Antonio, TX: Pearson.

Gottwald, S., & Dietrich, S. (2002). Therapy for school-age children who stutter. Workshop presented at the 2002 Stuttering Foundation of America Eastern Workshop. Boston, MA.

Guitar, B. (1998). *Stuttering: An integrated approach to its nature and treatment.* New York, NY: Lippincott, Williams, & Wilkins.

Hale, C. M., & Tager-Flusberg, H. (2005). Brief report: The relationship between discourse deficits and autism symptomology. *Journal of Autism and Developmental Disorders, 35*(4), 519–524.

Hallowell, E. M., & Ratey, J. J. (1994). *Driven to distraction: Recognizing and coping with attention deficit disorder from childhood through adulthood.* New York, NY: Pantheon.

Hartfield, K. N., & Conture, E. G. (2006). Effects of perceptual and conceptual similarity in lexical priming of young children who stutter: Preliminary findings. *Journal of Fluency Disorders, 31*(4), 303–324.

Healey, E. C., & Reid, R. (2003). ADHD and stuttering: A tutorial. *Journal of Fluency Disorders, 28*(2), 79–93.

Healey, K.T., Nelson, S., & Scaler Scott, K. (2015). Analysis of word-final dysfluencies in conversations of a child with autism: A treatment case study. *Procedia-Social and Behavioral Sciences, 193,* 147–152.

Heitman R, Asbjørnsen A, & Helland T. (2004). Attentional functions in speech fluency disorders. *Logopedics, Phoniatrics, Vocology, 29,*119–127.

Henry, L., Cornoldi, C., & Mahler, C. (2010). Special issues on working memory and executive functioning in individuals with intellectual disabilities. *Journal of Intellectual Disability Research, 54*(4), 293–294.

Hettinger Steiner, H., & Carr, M. (2003). Cognitive development in gifted children: Toward a more precise understanding of emerging differences in intelligence. *Educational Psychology Review, 15*(3), 215–246.

Hodson, B., & Paden, E. (1983). *Targeting intelligible speech: A phonological approach to remediation.* London, England: College Hill Press, Inc.

Hofmann, S. G. (2007). Cognitive factors that maintain social anxiety disorder: A comprehensive model and its treatment implications. *Cognitive Behaviour Therapy, 36*(4), 193–209.

Hollister, J., Van Horne, A. O., & Zebrowski, P. (2016). The relationship between grammatical development and disfluencies in preschool children who stutter and those who recover. *American Journal of Speech-Language Pathology,* 1–13.

Hua, A., & Major, N. (2016). Selective mutism. *Current Opinion in Pediatrics, 28*(1), 114–120.

International Dyslexia Association. (2017). *Dyslexia basics.* Retrieved from https://dyslexiaida.org/dyslexia-basics/

Ito, M., & Matsushima, E. (2016). Presentation of coping strategies associated with physical and mental health during health checkups. *Community Mental Health Journal, 53*(3), 297–305.

Joseph, R. M., Steele, S. D., Meyer, E., & Tager-Flusberg, H. (2005). Self-ordered pointing in children with autism: Failure to use verbal mediation in the service of working memory? *Neuropsychologia, 43*(10), 1400–1411.

Karniol, R. (1995). Stuttering, language, and cognition: A review and model of stuttering as suprasegmental sentence plan alignment (SPA). *Psychological Bulletin, 117,* 104–124.

Karrass, J., Walden, T. A., Conture, E. G., Graham, C. G., Arnold, H. S., Hartfield, K. N., & Schwenk, K. A. (2006). Relation of emotional reactivity and regulation to childhood stuttering. *Journal of Communication Disorders, 39*(6), 402–423.

Kent, R. D., & Vorperian, H. K. (2013). Speech impairment in Down syndrome: A review. *Journal of Speech, Language, and Hearing Research, 56*(1), 178–210.

Kidron, M., Scaler Scott, K., & Lozier, J. L. (2012, July). *Working memory in relation to children's cluttering symptoms in 3 speaking contexts.* Poster presented at the 7th World Congress on Fluency Disorders, Tours, France.

Klingberg, T. (2001). Cogmed. Retrieved from www.cogmed.com.

Kolk, H, & Postma, A. (1997). Stuttering as a covert repair phenomenon. In R. Curlee & G. Siegel (Eds.), *Nature and treatment of stuttering: New directions* (2nd ed., pp. 182–203). Boston, MA: Allyn & Bacon.

Koshino, H., Carpenter, P. A., Minshew, N. J., Cherkassky, V. L., & Keller, T. A., Just, M. A. (2005). Functional connectivity in an fMRI working memory task in high-functioning autism. *NeuroImage, 24,* 810–821.

Lake, J. K., Humphreys, J. R., & Cardy, S. (2011). Listener vs. speaker oriented aspects of speech: Studying the disfluencies of individuals with autism spectrum disorders. *Psychonomic Bulletin and Review, 18,* 135–140.

Lang, C., Nir, Z., Gothelf, A., Domachevsky, S., Ginton, L., Kushnir, J., & Gothelf, D. (2016). The outcome of children with selective mutism following cognitive behavioral intervention: a follow-up study. *European Journal of Pediatrics, 175*(4), 481.

Lebrun, Y., & Leleux, C. (1985). Acquired stuttering following right-brain damage in dextrals. *Journal of Fluency Disorders, 10,* 137–141.

Lebrun, Y., & Van Borsel, J. (1990). Final sound repetitions. *Journal of Fluency Disorders, 15,* 107–113.

Lee, J. K., & Orsillo, S. M. (2014). Investigating cognitive flexibility as a potential mechanism of mindfulness in generalized anxiety disorder. *Journal of Behavior Therapy and Experimental Psychiatry, 45*(1), 208–216.

Leslie, L., & Schudt Caldwell, J. (2017). *Qualitative Reading Inventory-6.* San Antonio, TX: Pearson.

Levelt, W. J. M. (1989). *Speaking: From intention to articulation.* Cambridge, MA: The MIT Press.

Lu, C., Chen, C., Ning, N., Ding, G., Guo, T., Peng, D., & Lin, C. (2010). The neural substrates for atypical planning and execution of word production in stuttering. *Experimental Neurology, 221*(1), 146–156.

Maas, E., Gildersleeve-Neumann, C., Jakielski, K. J., & Stoeckel, R. (2014). Motor-based intervention approaches in childhood apraxia of speech (cas). *Current Developmental Disorders Reports, 1*(3), 197–206. doi:10.1007/s40474-014-0016-4

McCauley, R. J., & Strand, E. (2008). Treatment of childhood apraxia of speech: Clinical decision making in the use of nonspeech oral motor exercises. *Seminars in Speech and Language, 29*(4), 284–293.

MacMillan, V., Kokolakis, A., Sheedy, S., & Packman, A. (2014). End-word dysfluencies in young children: A clinical report. *Folia Phoniatrica et Logopaedica, 66*(3), 115–125. doi:10.1159/000365247

Manassis, K., Oerbeck, B., & Overgaard, K. (2016). The use of medication in selective mutism: A systematic review. *European Child & Adolescent Psychiatry, 25*(6).

Markett, S., Bleek, B., Reuter, M., Prüss, H., Richardt, K., Müller, T., . . . Montag, C. (2016). Impaired motor inhibition in adults who stutter-evidence from speech-free stop-signal reaction time tasks. *Neuropsychologia, 91*, 444–450.

Martin, N.A. & Brownell, R. (2005). *Test of Auditory Processing Skills, Third Edition (TAPS-3).* Austin, TX: PRO-ED, Inc.

McAllister, J., & Kingston, M. (2005). Final part-word repetitions in school-age children: Two case studies. *Journal of Fluency Disorders, 30*(3), 255–267. doi:10.1016/j.jfludis.2005.05.005

McGill, M., Sussman, H., & Byrd, C. T. (2016). From grapheme to phonological output: Performance of adults who stutter on a word jumble task. *PLOS One.* doi.org/10.1371/journal.pone.0151107

McInnes, A., Fung, D., Manassis, K., Fiksenbaum, L., & Tannock, R. (2004). Narrative skills in children with selective mutism: An exploratory study. *American Journal of Speech-Language Pathology, 13*(4), 304–315.

Menzies, R. G., Onslow, M., Packman, A., & O'Brian, S. (2009). Cognitive behavior therapy for adults who stutter: A tutorial for speech-language pathologists. *Journal of Fluency Disorders, 34*(3), 187–200.

Minshew, N. J., & Williams, D. L. (2008). Brain-behavior connection in autism. In K. D. Buron & P. Wolfberg (Eds.), *Learners on the autism spectrum: Preparing highly qualified educators.* Shawnee, KS: Autism Asperger Publishing. Co.

Mowrer, D. E. (1987). Repetition of final consonants in the speech of a young child. *Journal of Speech and Hearing Disorders, 52*, 174–178.

Myers, F. L. (1992). Cluttering: A synergistic framework. In F. L. Myers, & K. O. St Louis (Eds.), *Cluttering: A clinical perspective* (pp. 71–84). Kibworth, England: Far Communications.

Myers, F. L. (2011). Treatment of cluttering: A cognitive-behavioral approach centered on rate control. In D. Ward & K. Scaler Scott (Eds.), *Cluttering: Research, Intervention and Education.* East Sussex, England: Psychology Press.

Myers, F. L., & Bradley, C. L. (1992). Clinical management of cluttering from a synergistic framework. In F. L. Myers & K. O. St. Louis (Eds.), *Cluttering: A clinical perspective* (pp. 85–106). Leicester, England: FAR Communications.

Myers, F. L. & St. Louis, K. O. (1996). Two youths who clutter, but is that the only similarity? *Journal of Fluency Disorders, 21*, 297–304.

Narad, M. E., Treble-Barna, A., Peugh, J., Yeates, K. O., Taylor, H. G., Stancin, T., & Wade, S. L. (2017). Recovery trajectories of executive functioning after pediatric TBI: A latent class growth modeling analysis. *The Journal of Head Trauma Rehabilitation, 32*(2), 98–106.

National Association for Gifted Children. (2010). *Redefining giftedness for a new century: Shifting the paradigm.* Washington, DC.

National Association for Gifted Children. (2017). A brief history of gifted and talented education. Retrieved from http://www.nagc.org/resources-publications/resources/gifted-education-us/brief-history-gifted-and-talented-education

National Association for Gifted Children. (2017). Definitions of giftedness. Retrieved from http://www.nagc.org/resources-publications/resources/definitions-giftedness

National Center for Learning Disabilities. (2013, April). LD defined: Specific learning disabilities. Retrieved from www.ld.org

National Society for the Gifted & Talented. (2017). Giftedness defined. Retrieved from https://www.nsgt.org/giftedness-defined/#1

Natke, U., Sandrieser, P., Van Ark, M., Pietrowsky, R., & Kalveram, K. T. (2004). Linguistic stress, within-word position, and grammatical class in relation to early childhood stuttering. *Journal of Fluency Disorders*, 1–21.

Nippold, M. A. (1990). Concomitant speech and language disorders in stuttering children. *Journal of Speech and Hearing Disorders, 55*, 51–60.

Nowakowski, M. E., Tasker, S. L., Cunningham, C. E., McHolm, A. E., Edison, S., St. Pierre, J., . . . Schmidt, L. A. (2011). Joint attention in parent-child dyads involving children with selective mutism: A comparison between anxious and typically developing children. *Child Psychiatry & Human Development, 42*, 78–92.

Ntourou, K., Conture, E. G., & Walden, T. A. (2013). Emotional reactivity and regulation in preschool-age children who stutter. *Journal of Fluency Disorders, 38*(3) 1–15.

Ochs, E., & Solomon, O. (2004). Introduction: Discourse and autism. *Discourse Studies, 6*(2), 139–146.

Osborne, C. (2004). A child with atypical stuttering: A case study. *Fluency and Fluency Disorders*, 3–6.

Ozonoff, S., Pennington, B. F., & Rogers, S. J. (1991). Executive function deficits in high-functioning autistic individuals: Relationship to theory of mind. *Journal of Child Psychology and Psychiatry, 32*(7), 1081–1105.

Packman, A., Onslow, M., Richard, F., & van Doorn, J. (1996). Syllabic stress and variability: A model of stuttering. *Clinical Linguistics and Phonetics, 10*, 235–263.

Paden, E. P., Yairi, E., & Ambrose, N. G. (1999). Early childhood stuttering II: Initial status of phonological abilities. *Journal of Speech, Language, and Hearing Research, 42*, 1113–1124.

Park, J., & Moghaddam, B. (2017). Impact of anxiety on prefrontal cortex encoding of cognitive flexibility. *Neuroscience, 345*, 193–202.

Paul, R. & Norbury, C. (2012). *Language disorders from infancy through adolescence: Listening, speaking, reading, writing, and communicating* (4th ed.). St Louis, MO: Elsevier, Mosby.

Pearson Education, Inc. (2016). Cogmed Working Memory Training Program. Minneapolis, MN.

Pelczarski, K. M., & Yaruss, J. S. (2014). Phonological encoding of young children who stutter. *Journal of Fluency Disorders, 39*, 12–24.

Pelczarski, K. M., & Yaruss, J. S. (2016). Phonological memory in young children who stutter. *Journal of Communication Disorders, 62*, 54–66.

Pellowski, M. W., & Conture, E. G. (2005). Lexical priming in picture naming of young children who do and do not stutter. *Journal of Speech, Language, and Hearing Research, 48*(2), 278–294.

Perkins, W. H., Kent, R. D., & Curlee, R. F. (1991). A theory of neuropsycholinguistic function in stuttering. *Journal of Speech and Hearing Research, 34*, 734–752.

Piispala, J., Kallio, M., Bloigu, R., & Jansson-Verkaslo, E. (2016). Delayed N2 response in Go condition in a visual Go/Nogo ERP study in children who stutter. *Journal of Fluency Disorders, 48*, 16–26.

Plexico, L., Cleary, J. E., McAlpine, A., & Plumb, A. M. (2010). Disfluency characteristics observed in young children with autism spectrum disorders: A preliminary report. *Perspectives on Fluency and Fluency Disorders*, 42–50.

Plexico, L., Manning, W. H., & DiLollo, A. (2005). A phenomenological understanding of successful stuttering management. *Journal of Fluency Disorders, 30*, 1–22.

Plexico, L. W., Manning, W. H., & DiLollo, A. (2010). Client perceptions of effective and ineffective therapeutic alliances during treatment for stuttering. *Journal of Fluency Disorders, 35,* 333-354.

Postma, A., & Kolk, H. (1993). The Covert Repair Hypothesis: Prearticulatory repair processes in normal and stuttered disfluencies. *Journal of Speech and Hearing Research, 36,* 472-487.

Power, A. J., Colling, L. J., Mead, N., Barnes, L., & Goswami, U. (2016). Neural encoding of the speech envelope by children with developmental dyslexia. *Brain & Language, 160,* 1-10.

Raphael, L. J., Bakker, K., Myers, F., & St. Louis, K. O. (2010, April). Spectrographic characteristics of cluttered speech rate (pp. 162-170). Proceedings of the First World Conference on Cluttering. Katarino, Bulgaria. Retrieved from http://associations.missouristate.edu/ICA

Richer, L., Lachance, L., & Côté, A. (2016). Relationship between age and psychopathological manifestations in school-age children with an intellectual disability: The role of executive functioning. *DADD Online Journal, 3*(1), 181-200.

Riley, G. D. (2009). *Stuttering Severity Instrument, Fourth Edition (SSI-4).* Austin, TX: PRO-ED, Inc.

Robertson, C., & Salter, W. (2007). *The Phonological Awareness Test 2.* Austin, TX: PRO-ED, Inc.

Roedell, W. (1984). Vulnerabilities of highly gifted children. *Roeper Review,* 127-130.

Rudmin, F. (1984). Parent's report of stress and articulation oscillation as factors in preschooler's dysfluencies. *Journal of Fluency Disorders, 9*(1), 85-87. doi:10.1016/0094-730X(84)90009-3

Sasisekaran, J. (2014). Exploring the link between stuttering and phonology: A review and implications for treatment. *Seminars in Speech and Language, 35*(2), 95-113. doi: 10.1055/s-0034-1371754

Scaler Scott, K. (2011). Cluttering and autism spectrum disorders. In D. Ward & K. Scaler Scott (Eds.). *Cluttering: Research, Intervention and Education.* East Sussex, England: Psychology Press.

Scaler Scott, K. (2014). Dysfluency in autism spectrum disorders. *Procedia-Social and Behavioral Sciences,* 2-7.

Scaler Scott, K., Block, S., Reardon-Reeves, N., Healey, K., Kerestes, K., LaRussa, R., . . . Kidron, M. (2013, Nov.). Disfluency in autism spectrum disorders: Treatment outcomes and what they mean for school-based speech-language pathologists. Seminar presented at the Annual Convention of the American Speech-Language Hearing Association, Chicago, IL.

Scaler Scott, K., Bossler, R., & Veneziale, A. (2015, Nov.). Response inhibition in cluttering. Poster presented at the Annual Convention of the American Speech Language Hearing Association, Denver, CO.

Scaler Scott, K., Bossler, R., Veneziale, A., Croasdale, S., & Irr, A. (2016, April). Response inhibition in cluttering: Next steps in analysis. Poster presented at the Annual Convention of the Pennsylvania Speech-Language Hearing Association, Pittsburgh, PA.

Scaler Scott, K., Grossman, H. L., Abendroth, K. J., Tetnowski, J. A., & Damico, J. S. (2007). Asperger syndrome and attention deficit disorder: Clinical disfluency analysis. In J. Au-Yeung & M. M. Leahy (Eds.). *Research, treatment, and self-help in fluency disorders: New horizons. Proceedings of the Fifth World Congress on Fluency Disorders.* Dublin, Ireland: International Fluency Association.

Scaler Scott, K., Harris, A., & St. Louis, K. O. (2013, Nov.). Spectrographic features and SLP diagnoses of one sample of cluttering. Poster presented at the Annual Convention of the American Speech-Language Hearing Association, Chicago, IL.

Scaler Scott, K., Kidron, M., & Lozier, J. (2012, Nov.). Comparison of cluttering symptoms in children in three speaking contexts. Poster presented at the Annual Convention of the American Speech-Language Hearing Association, Atlanta, GA.

Scaler Scott, K., Nelson, S., Block, S., Reeves, N., Kidron, M., Healey, K., . . . Tokach, S. (2014, April). Schools-based training model for treating disfluencies in children with autism. Poster presented at the Annual Convention of the Pennsylvania Speech-Language Hearing Association, Pittsburgh, PA.

Scaler Scott, K., Reeves, N., Block, S., & Kidron, M., & Lozier, J. (2011, Nov.). Training SLPs to treat fluency disorders in students with ASDs. Seminar presented at the Annual Convention of the American Speech-Language Hearing Association, San Diego, CA.

Scaler Scott, K., & Sisskin, V. (2007). Speech disfluency in autism spectrum disorders, Part two: Clinical problem solving for pervasive developmental disorder, not otherwise specified and Asperger syndrome. Online conference at the Tenth Annual International Stuttering Awareness Day (ISAD).

Scaler Scott, K., & St. Louis, K. O. (2011). Consumer issues: Self-help for people with cluttering. In D. Ward & K. Scaler Scott (Eds.), *Cluttering: Research, Intervention and Education.* East Sussex, England: Psychology Press.

Scaler Scott, K., Sutkowski, S., Tokach, S., & Leiman, B. (2015, Nov.). Communicative contexts that elicit word final disfluencies. Seminar presented at the Annual Convention of the American Speech-Language Hearing Association, Denver, CO.

Scaler Scott, K., Sutkowski, S., Tokach, S., Leiman, B., Irr, A., Veneziale, A., . . . Giacumbo, K. (in preparation). Atypical disfluency in school-age children: Cognitive-linguistic profiles.

Scaler Scott, K., Tetnowski, J. A., Flaitz, J., & Yaruss, J. S. (2014, Jan-Feb). Preliminary study of disfluency in school-age children with autism. *International Journal of Language and Communication Disorders, 49*(1), 75-89.

Scaler Scott, K., & Ward, D. (2013). *Managing cluttering: A comprehensive guidebook of activities.* Austin, TX: Pro-Ed, Inc.

Scaler Scott, K., Ward, D., & St. Louis, K. O. (2010). Paul: Treatment of cluttering in a school-age child. In S. Chabon and E. Cohn (Eds.), *The communication disorders casebook: Learning by example* (pp. 261-272). Boston, MA: Pearson.

Schleef, E. (2005). Gender, power, discipline, and context: On the sociolinguistic variation of okay, right, like, and you know in English academic discourse. *Texas Linguistic Forum, 48,* 177-186.

Scientific Learning Corporation (1998). Fast ForWord Language Series. Retrieved from www.scilearn.com.

Semel, E., Wiig, E. H., & Secord, W.A. (1995). *Clinical Evaluation of Language Fundamentals, Third Edition (CELF-3).* San Antonio, TX: Pearson.

Shulman, L. S. (1986). Those who understand: Knowledge growth in teaching. *Educational Researcher, 15*(2), 4-14.

Singer, B. D., & Bashir, A. S. (1999). What are executive functions and self-regulations and what do they have to do with language-learning disorders? *Language, Speech, and Hearing Services in Schools, 30,* 265-273.

Sisskin, V. (2006). Speech disfluency in Asperger's syndrome: Two cases of interest. *Perspectives on Fluency and Fluency Disorders, 16*(2), 12-14.

Sisskin, V., & Wasilus, S. (2014, May). Lost in the literature, but not the caseload: Working with atypical disfluency from theory to practice. *Seminars in Speech and Language, 35*(2), 144-152.

Smith, A. (1990a). Toward a comprehensive theory of stuttering: A commentary. *Journal of Speech and Hearing Disorders, 55,* 398-401.

Smith, A. (1990b). Factors in the etiology of stuttering. *American Speech-Language-Hearing Association Reports, Research Needs in Stuttering: Roadblocks and Future Directions, 18,* 39-47.

Smith, A., & Kelly, E. (1997). Stuttering: A dynamic, multifactorial model. In R. F. Curlee & G. M. Siegel (Eds.), *Nature and treatment of stuttering: New directions* (2nd ed., pp. 204-217). Needham Heights, MD: Allyn & Bacon.

Sonneville-Koedoot, C., Stolk, E., Rietveld, T., & Franken, M. C. (2015). Direct versus indirect treatment for preschool children who stutter: The restart randomized trial. *PLOS One,* 1-17.

Stansfield, J. (1995).Word-final disfluencies in adults with learning difficulties. *Journal of Fluency Disorders, 20,* 1-10.

Starkweather, C. W. (1987). *Fluency and stuttering.* Englewood Cliffs, NJ: Prentice-Hall.

Stewart, C. R., Sanchez, S. S., Gronesko, E. L., Brown, C. M., Chen, C. P., Keehn, B., . . . Müller, R. A. (2015). Sensory symptoms and processing of nonverbal auditory and visual stimuli in children with autism spectrum disorders. *Journal of Autism and Developmental Disorders, 46*(5), 1590–1601.

St. John, T., Estes, A. M., Dager, S. R., Kostopoulos, P., Wolff, J. J., Pandey, J., . . . Piven, J. (2016). Emerging executive functioning and motor development in infants at high and low risk for autism spectrum disorder. *Frontiers in Psychology, 7*, 1–12.

St. Louis, K. O. (1992). On defining cluttering. In F. L. Myers & K. O. St. Louis (Eds.), *Cluttering: A clinical perspective*. Kibworth, England: Far Communications.

St. Louis, K. O. (1996). A tabular summary of cluttering subjects in the special edition. *Journal of Fluency Disorders, 21*, 337–343.

St. Louis, K. O., Goranova, E., Georgieva, D., Coskun, M., Filatova, Y., & McCaffrey, E. (2010, April). Public awareness of cluttering: USA, Bulgaria, Turkey, Russia (pp. 180–189). Proceedings of the First World Conference on Cluttering. Katarino, Bulgaria. Retrieved from http://associations.missouristate.edu/ICA.

St. Louis, K. O., Myers, F., Bakker, K., & Raphael, L. (2007). Understanding and treating cluttering. In Conture, E. & Curlee, R. (Eds.), *Stuttering and related disorders of fluency* (3rd ed., pp. 297–325). New York, NY: Thieme.

St. Louis, K. O., Raphael, L. J., Myers, F. L., & Bakker, K. (2003). Cluttering updated. The ASHA Leader. Retrieved from http://leader.pubs.asha.org/article.aspx?articleid=2292318

St. Louis, K. O., & Schulte, K. (2011). Defining cluttering: The lowest common denominator. In D. Ward & K. Scaler Scott (Eds.), *Cluttering: Research, Intervention and Education*. East Sussex, England: Psychology Press.

Strand, E. A., Stoeckel, R., & Baas, B. Treatment of severe childhood apraxia of speech: A treatment efficacy study. *Journal of Medical Speech-Language Pathology, 14*, 297–307.

Sutkowski, S., Scaler Scott, K., Kisenwether, J., Thomas, K., & Anson, D. (2016, Nov.). Duration analysis of silent intervals in word-final disfluencies. Poster presented at the Annual Convention of the American Speech Language Hearing Association, Philadelphia, PA.

Sutkowski, S., Tokach, S., & Scaler Scott, K. (2015). Language profiles and linguistic contexts related to word final disfluencies in school-age children. Poster presented at the Annual Convention of the American Speech-Language-Hearing Association. Denver, CO.

Swift, M. C., Jones, M., O'Brian, S., Onslow, M., Packman, A., & Menzies, R. (2016). Parent verbal contingencies during the Lidcombe Program: Observations and statistical modeling of the treatment process. *Journal of Fluency Disorders, 47*, 13–26.

Tetnowski, J., Richels, C., Shenker, R., Sisskin, V., & Wolk, L. (2012). When the diagnosis is dual. *ASHA Leader*, 10–13.

Thurik, R., Khedhaouria, A., Torres, O., & Verheul, I. (2016). ADHD symptoms and entrepreneurial orientation of small firm owners. *Applied Psychology: An International Review, 65*(3), 568–586.

Tiger, R. J., Irvine, T. L., & Reis, R. P. (1980). Cluttering as a complex of learning disabilities. *Language, Speech, and Hearing Services in Schools*, 3–14.

Usler, E., & Weber-Fox, C. (2015). Neurodevelopment for syntactic processing distinguishes childhood stuttering recovery versus persistence. *Journal of Neurodevelopmental Disorders, 7*(4), 1–21.

Van Borsel, J., (2011). Cluttering and Down syndrome. In D. Ward & K. Scaler Scott (Eds.). *Cluttering: Research, Intervention and Education*. East Sussex, England: Psychology Press.

Van Borsel, J., Geirnaert, E., & Van Coster, R. (2005). Another case of word-final disfluencies. *Folia Phoniatrica et Logopaedica, 57*(3), 148–162.

Van Borsel, J., & Tetnowski, J. A. (2007). Fluency disorders in genetic syndromes. *Journal of Fluency Disorders, 32*(4), 279–296.

Van Borsel, J., Van Coster, R., & Van Lierd, K. (1996). Repetitions in final position in a nine-year-old boy with focal brain damage. *Journal of Fluency Disorders, 21*, 137–146.

Van Borsel, J., & Vandermeulen, A. (2008). Cluttering in Down syndrome. *Folia Phoniatrica et Logopaedica, 60*(6), 312–317.

Van Riper, C. (1973). *The Treatment of Stuttering*. Englewood Cliffs, NJ: Prentice-Hall

Van Zaalen, Y., & Reichel, I. (2015). *Cluttering: Current views on its nature, diagnosis, and treatment*. Bloomington, IN: iUniverse.

Van Zaalen, Y., Wijnen, F., & Dejonckere, P. (2011a). The assessment of cluttering: Rationale, tasks, and interpretation. In D. Ward & K. Scaler Scott (Eds.). *Cluttering: Research, Intervention and Education*. East Sussex, England: Psychology Press.

Van Zaalen, Y., Wijnen, F., & Dejonckere, P. (2011b). Cluttering and learning disabilities. In D. Ward & K. Scaler Scott (Eds.). *Cluttering: Research, Intervention and Education*. East Sussex, England: Psychology Press.

Vanryckeghem, M., & Brutten, G. J. (2006). *KiddyCAT: Communication attitude test for preschool and kindergarten children who stutter*. San Diego, CA: Plural Publishing, Inc.

Veneziale, A., Irr, A., Scaler Scott, K., Gurtizen, E., & Leiman, B. (2017, March). Conversation analysis: Determining the function of word-final disfluencies. Poster presented at the Annual Convention of the Pennsylvania Speech-Language Hearing Association, Harrisburg, PA.

Viana, A. G., Beidel, D. C., & Rabian, B. (2009). Selective mutism: A review and integration of the last 15 years. *Clinical Psychology Review, 29*(1), 57–67.

Wagner, R. K., Torgesen, J. K., Rashotte, C. A., & Pearson, N.A. (2013). *Comprehensive Test of Phonological Processing, Second Edition (CTOPP-2)*. Austin, TX: PRO-ED, Inc.

Ward, D., Connally, E. L., Pliatsikas, C., Bretherton-Furness, J., & Watkins, K. E. (2015). The neurological underpinnings of cluttering: Some initial findings. *Journal of Fluency Disorders, 43*, 1–16.

Ward, D., & Scaler Scott, K. (Eds.). (2011). *Cluttering: A handbook of research, intervention, and education*. London, England: Psychology Press.

Watson, S. M. R., Gable, R. A., & Morin, L. L. (2016). The role of executive functions in classroom instruction of students with learning disabilities. *International Journal of School and Cognitive Psychology, 3*(1), 1–5.

Webb, J. T. (1993). Nurturing social-emotional development of gifted children. In K. A. Heller, F. J. Monks, & A. H., Passow (Eds.), *Research and development of giftedness and talent*. New York, NY: Pergamon.

Weiss, D. (1964). *Cluttering*. Englewood Cliffs, NJ: Prentice-Hall.

White, H., & Shah, P. (2006). Uninhibited imaginations: Creativity in adults with attention-deficit/hyperactivity disorder. *Personality and Individual Difference, 40*, 1121–1131.

Widerholt, J.L., & Bryant, B.R. (2012). *Gray Oral Reading Tests, Fifth Edition (GORT-5)*. Austin, TX: PRO-ED, Inc.

Williams, D. F. (2016). Putting thoughts into words: Verbal encoding in autism spectrum disorders [Powerpoint slides]. Retrieved from Pennsylvania Speech-Language Hearing Association.

Williams, K. T. (2007). *Expressive Vocabulary Test, Second Edition (EVT-2)*. San Antonio, TX: Pearson.

Williams, M., & Kabat-Zinn, J. (2013). *Mindfulness: Diverse perspectives on its meaning, origins, and applications*. New York, NY: Routledge.

Wright, L., & Ayre, A. (2000). *WASSP: Wright and Ayre stuttering self-rating profile*. Bicester, England: Speechmark.

Wu, J. C., Maguire, G., Riley, G., Lee, A., Keator, D., Tang, C., . . . Najafi, A. (1997). Increased dopamine activity associated with stuttering. *Neuroreport, 8*(3), 767–770.

Yairi, E., & Ambrose, N. (1992). A longitudinal study of stuttering in children: A preliminary report. *Journal of Speech and Hearing Research, 35*, 755–760.

Yairi, E., Ambrose, N., & Cox, N. (1996). Genetics of Stuttering: A Critical Review. *Journal of Speech and Hearing Research, 39*, 771-784.

Yairi, E., & Ambrose, N. (2013). Epidemiology of stuttering: 21st century advances. *Journal of Fluency Disorders, 38*(2), 66–87.

Yaruss, J. S. (1998). Real-time analysis of speech fluency: Procedures and reliability training. *American Journal of Speech-Language Pathology, 7*(2), 25–37.

Yaruss, J. S., Coleman, C., & Hammer, D. (2006). Treating preschool children who stutter: Description and preliminary evaluation of a family-focused treatment approach. *Language, Speech, and Hearing Services in Schools, 37*, 118–136.

Yaruss, J. S., & Quesal, R. W. (2006). Overall assessment of the speaker's experience of stuttering (OASES): Documenting multiple outcomes in stuttering treatment. *Journal of Fluency Disorders, 31*, 90–115.

Yaruss, J. S., & Quesal, R. W., & Coleman, C. (2006). Overall assessment of the speaker's experience of stuttering (OASES). Stuttering Therapy Resources. Retrieved from www.stutteringtherapyresources.com

Ylvisaker, M., Turkstra, L., Coehlo, C., Yorkston, K., Kennedy, M., Sohlberg, M. M., & Avery, J. (2007). Behavioural interventions for children and adults with behaviour disorders after TBI: A systematic review of the evidence. *Brain Injury, 21*(8), 769–805.

Zhang, W., Fan, L., & Jiang, Y. P. (2015). *Medicine and biopharmaceutical*. Japan: World Scientific.

# INDEX

language-based activities with fluency focus
  for, 116–124
language development differences and, 179
with learning differences, 110
multifactorial etiology of, 11–12
myths about, 13
repetitions, 5
secondary behaviors of, 5–6
with selective mutism, 163
self-monitoring and, 54
task persistence and, 66
word retrieval and, 61–62
stuttering blocks, versus mid-word insertions,
  22–23
stuttering-like disfluencies, 5
  in intellectual disability population, 85
stuttering modification, 88–90
syllable stress, abnormal, 22
syntactic processing deficits, 176

talent, definition of, 175. *See also* gifted and
  talented population
task persistence, 66–67
  in gifted and talented population, 177–178,
    179
  in intellectual disability population, 88
  in learning disability population, 112
teacher role, 88, 91, 101
  for ADHD population, 142
teamwork, in treating concomitant disorders,
  44–45
thoughts, changing, 173
time management, in ADHD, 137
Tourette syndrome, 10, 36
transitions between sounds, building, 75–76
treatment flexibility, 39–41
Turner syndrome, 36

verbal communication strategies, with selective
  mutism, 167
video retell transcript, 33
visual organizers, in autism spectrum disorder, 149
visual processing disorders, 109

weak syllable deletion, 75
word-final disfluencies, 1, 9, 10
  cognitive components of, 11
  in gifted and talented population, 180–182
  in intellectual disability population, 85–86
  in learning disability population, 114
  phonological encoding and, 60
  response inhibition and, 58
  with selective mutism, 163
  self-monitoring and, 55
  working memory and, 16
word-final repetitions, 9
  with insertions, 10
word finding difficulties, 23–24
word-medial repetitions, 9, 10–11
word retrieval, 61–63
  activities targeting, 150, 155
  activities with fluency focus for, 116
  in atypical disfluencies, 93
  in learning disability population, 114
  with selective mutism, 164
  with stuttering, 38–39
word study, 126–127
working memory, 56–57
  activities targeting, 150
  in ADHD, 134–135
  in atypical disfluencies, 16, 93
  in autism spectrum disorder, 149
  cluttering and, 51
  in gifted and talented population, 179–180
  in intellectual disability population, 88
working memory game, 156

Printed in the United States
by Baker & Taylor Publisher Services